Psychiatry - Theory, Applications and Treatments

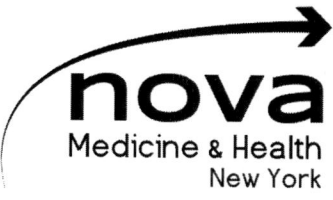

Medicine & Health
New York

Psychiatry - Theory, Applications and Treatments

Humanist Psychiatry, 2nd Edition
Nash N. Boutros, MD (Editor)
2022. ISBN: 978-1-68507-501-9 (Softcover)
2022. ISBN: 978-1-68507-544-6 (eBook)

**Obsessive-Compulsive Disorder:
Symptoms, Therapy and Clinical Challenges**
Jeffrey L. Nelson (Editor)
2021. ISBN: 978-1-68507-310-7 (Softcover)
2021. ISBN: 978-1-68507-326-8 (eBook)

Perinatal Depression
Jennifer Lynn Barkin, Marta Serati
and Massimiliano Buoli (Editors)
2020. ISBN: 978-1-53617-301-7 (eBook)

Forensic Psychiatry and Ethical Approaches in Legal Issues
Nursen Turan Yurtsever (Editor)
2021. ISBN: 978-1-53619-530-9 (Hardcover)
2021. ISBN: 978-1-53619-606-1 (eBook)

Innovations in Psychiatry
Panagiota Korenis, MD, Souparno Mitra, MD
and Urmi Chaudhuri (Editors)
2021. ISBN: 978-1-53619-365-7 (Hardcover)
2021. ISBN: 978-1-53619-438-8 (eBook)

More information about this series can be found at
https://novapublishers.com/product-category/series/psychiatry-theory-applications-and-treatments/

Charles L. Burgess
Editor

Understanding Psychotic Disorders

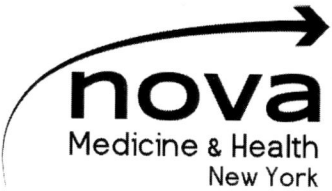

Copyright © 2022 by Nova Science Publishers, Inc.

All rights reserved. No part of this book may be reproduced, stored in a retrieval system or transmitted in any form or by any means: electronic, electrostatic, magnetic, tape, mechanical photocopying, recording or otherwise without the written permission of the Publisher.

We have partnered with Copyright Clearance Center to make it easy for you to obtain permissions to reuse content from this publication. Simply navigate to this publication's page on Nova's website and locate the "Get Permission" button below the title description. This button is linked directly to the title's permission page on copyright.com. Alternatively, you can visit copyright.com and search by title, ISBN, or ISSN.

For further questions about using the service on copyright.com, please contact:
Copyright Clearance Center
Phone: +1-(978) 750-8400   Fax: +1-(978) 750-4470   E-mail: info@copyright.com.

NOTICE TO THE READER

The Publisher has taken reasonable care in the preparation of this book, but makes no expressed or implied warranty of any kind and assumes no responsibility for any errors or omissions. No liability is assumed for incidental or consequential damages in connection with or arising out of information contained in this book. The Publisher shall not be liable for any special, consequential, or exemplary damages resulting, in whole or in part, from the readers' use of, or reliance upon, this material. Any parts of this book based on government reports are so indicated and copyright is claimed for those parts to the extent applicable to compilations of such works.

Independent verification should be sought for any data, advice or recommendations contained in this book. In addition, no responsibility is assumed by the Publisher for any injury and/or damage to persons or property arising from any methods, products, instructions, ideas or otherwise contained in this publication.

This publication is designed to provide accurate and authoritative information with regard to the subject matter covered herein. It is sold with the clear understanding that the Publisher is not engaged in rendering legal or any other professional services. If legal or any other expert assistance is required, the services of a competent person should be sought. FROM A DECLARATION OF PARTICIPANTS JOINTLY ADOPTED BY A COMMITTEE OF THE AMERICAN BAR ASSOCIATION AND A COMMITTEE OF PUBLISHERS.

Additional color graphics may be available in the e-book version of this book.

Library of Congress Cataloging-in-Publication Data

ISBN: 979-8-88697-336-5

Published by Nova Science Publishers, Inc. † New York

Contents

Preface vii

Chapter 1   **The Spectrum of Negative Symptoms across Schizophrenia and Affective Psychosis: Contribution to Prognosis** 1
Petar S. Popov, Stefan P. Popov
and Drozdstoy S. Stoyanov

Chapter 2   **Propriety of Proof of Concept (PoC) Trials in Interactive Social Cognition Interventions: A Program Summary of Mentalization-Based Group Therapy - *Interactional* (MBGT-*i*)** 35
Killorin Riddell and Monty Clouse

Chapter 3   **Psychotic Disorders and Contributing Factors in Adolescence** 61
Carmen Cendrero-Luengo,
María Jiménez-Palomares,
Juan Rodríguez-Mansilla,
María Jesús Rodríguez-Mansilla,
María Trinidad Rodríguez-Domínguez
and Elisa María Garrido-Ardila

Chapter 4   **Narcissistic Personality Wounds in Music Therapists** 77
Antonia de la Torre-Rísquez,
Maria Isabel Ramos-Fuentes,
Elisa María Garrido-Ardila,
María Jiménez-Palomares,
Manuel Sequera-Martín
and Juan Rodríguez-Mansilla

Bibliography 87

Index 199

Functional abnormalities of the cerebellum in schizophrenia patients are investigated by the voxel-wise data-driven method, resting-state functional magnetic resonance imaging data. A decreased resting-state functional connectivity (rsFCD) is present in the right hemisphere. rsFC is increased between that cerebellar region and the prefrontal cortex and subcortical nuclei. This suggests that maybe the abnormality of the cerebellar functional connectivity can be a neural mechanism of schizophrenia. Anatomically, the cerebellum is a heterogeneous structure and is divided into vermal and hemispheric subregions. Task-based neuroimaging suggests that the cerebellum subregions are involved in many important functions like motor-related processing, cognitive and affective processing (Zhuo et al. 2018).

There are brain structures like default mode network (DMN) and executive control network (ECN) which are abnormal in schizophrenia patients. The locus coeruleus (LC) noradrenaline (NE) system plays a major role in the occurrence of positive and negative symptoms of schizophrenia. There is an increased Blood oxygen level development (BOLD) activation in the LC in patients with Schizophrenia. The core hubs of the ECN system are the dorsolateral prefrontal cortex, ventrolateral prefrontal cortex, parietal cortex, and striatum. In patients with Schizophrenia, there are working memory impairments and ECN dysfunctions. The main hub of the DMN which is the PCC is deactivated in healthy persons and schizophrenia patients. Data exist for an increased BOLD activation in ECN and DMN BOLD deactivation (Suttkus et al. 2021).

It is not so easy to make the differential diagnosis between SZ and other Psychiatric disorders, particularly Mood disorders. One study tries to distinguish these disorders at the beginning, or at the early years of their development by using four morphometric measures – gyrification, cortical thickness, whole-brain grey matter, and grey matter volume (Madeira et al. 2020). An increased volume of the right globus pallidus and decreased gyrification of the right inferior frontal gyrus in patients with SZ and a divergent gyrification of the left supramarginal gyrus in BPD were also found. An increased volume of the globus pallidus was present at the early stages of disease in schizophrenic patients. As a result, changes in gyrification can be used as a biomarker in patients with BPD.

In schizophrenia, there is a decreased intrinsic functional connectivity between prefrontal-limbic cortices and thalamic nuclei. At the same time, an increased iFC between primary-sensorimotor cortices and thalamic nuclei exists. There is an inter-correlated hypoconnectivity between the prefrontal-limbic salience network and thalamus, striatum, and pallidum as well as a hyperconnectivity between the auditory-sensorimotor network and the same subcortical structures. SAL cortico-subcortical hypoconnectivity was linked to cognitive impairment. It follows from all this that there is a relationship between distinct cortico-subcortical hypo-hyperconnectivity and different symptoms. SAL hypoconnectivity with thalamus striatum and pallidum is specifically associated with cognitive impairments in terms of reduced verbal fluency, but not psychotic symptoms measured by the PANSS+ scale. Other studies suggest a correlation between reduced prefrontal-thalamic structural connectivity and working memory in patients with schizophrenia (Avram et al. 2018).

Although cognitive deficits are common in schizophrenia the neural mechanisms behind them need more research. Structures like the dorsolateral prefrontal cortex (DLPFC), inferior frontal gyrus, hippocampus, and white matter are associated with cognitive impairment, executive functioning, working memory, verbal memory, verbal fluency, and so on. Global cognition is associated with brain structures like DLPFC, IFG, hippocampus, and white matter, and these brain structures are crucial for cognitive functioning through distinct support of executive functions (Jirsaraie et al. 2018).

Reduced prefrontal-thalamic and increased sensorimotor-thalamic functional connectivity is present in schizophrenia patients. Cognitive deficits are mainly related to the functional connectivity of the thalamic PFC subregions, which correspond closely to the thalamic mediodorsal nucleus. Other studies find reduced structural connectivity between lateral PFC and the mediodorsal nucleus. Mediodorsal thalamus refers to working memory and attentional control - thalamic PFC subregions play the main role in cognitive symptoms of schizophrenia. There is a negative correlation between thalamic functional connectivity with sensorimotor regions and higher cognitive functions. As an example during the sequential finger-tapping task, there was a reduced activation of the sensorimotor cortices. Decreased connectivity of the cerebellum with the thalamic PFC subregion is in positive correlation with cognitive function in schizophrenia. The dysfunction of the thalamus might act as a mediator in the synchronized activity between the cerebellum and prefrontal cortex in schizophrenia patients. Also, negative symptoms of deficit schizophrenia are positively related to hyperconnectivity between the thalamus and sensorimotor cortex (Chen et al. 2019).

Cognitive functions like working memory, cognitive flexibility, and inhibition are impaired in schizophrenia. Cognitive impairment can be a predictor of functional outcomes. Reduced anatomical connectivity between the PFC and thalamus connectivity in schizophrenia is related to impaired executive function. Various studies support the idea of a correlation between the lateral PFC - thalamic connectivity and working memory. Connectivity is reduced in the orbitofrontal cortex, but not in lateral and medial PFC Resting-state fMRI investigations find a reduced functional connectivity between the PFC and thalamus in schizophrenia (Giraldo-Chica et al. 2018).

Most Schizophrenia patients show cognitive impairment and the reason can be damage to brain regions. The hippocampus - a brain structure involved in memory and mood function shows impairment in schizophrenia. Patients with schizophrenia have a wide range of cognitive and mood problems, including working memory and executive functions deficits. Neuroimaging techniques suggest an abnormality of the hippocampus in schizophrenia, particularly gray matter volume loss in the hippocampus VBM shows reduced gray matter volume in the parahippocampal gyrus, inferior temporal gyrus, and insular cortex (Singh et al. 2018).

The role of white matter microstructure for many cognitive measures is very important and crucial. The whole-brain white matter is significantly mediated by working memory and processing speed. The latter significantly mediates fractional anisotropy – to working memory effects. The prolonged development of associative white matter regions may affect processing speed and working memory in schizophrenia patients. In this way schizophrenia is both a neurodevelopmental and neurodegenerative disorder (Kochunov et al. 2017).

Working memory task performance is associated with functional connectivity. Working memory is associated with many regions – the dorsolateral prefrontal cortex, the ventrolateral prefrontal cortex, encompassing the inferior frontal gyrus, as well as posterior parietal regions, including the intraparietal sulcus and temporoparietal junction (Wylie et al. 2019).

Deficits in executive function and attention are linked to dysfunction of the dorsolateral prefrontal cortex. The DLPFC can be divided into two parts – anterior and posterior. Reduced corticostriatal connectivity is a trait characteristic in schizophrenia patients. DLPFC is involved in high-order control processes of motor behavior such as attention and subsequent behavioral adjustments. Lower activation in the posterior parietal cortices together with decreased frontoparietal functional connectivity during a working memory task can be a serious risk factor for childhood-onset of schizophrenia (Chechko et al. 2018).

There is a correlation between cognitive deficits and white matter aging in schizophrenia patients. Worsened performance of working memory and processing speed also has a relationship with the age of the patients (Wang et al. 2021).

Affected brain regions in schizophrenia patients induce dysfunction of the working memory. The BOLD effect is widely used in fMRI studies, representing an increased inflow of oxygenated blood as an answer to brain activity in a particular region. Different types of paradigms such as visual tasks and auditory oddballs are used to find the pattern of functioning of the brain during different cognitive processes. Functional activation of particular brain regions was observed – cerebellum, inferior temporal gyrus, superior temporal gyrus, superior frontal gyrus, insula, amygdala, thalamus, occipital lobe, and hippocampus. Changes in the Heschl gyrus region like grey matter atrophy were noticed. Inferior temporal gyrus, superior temporal gyrus, insula region, and superior frontal gyrus were also affected (Chatterjee et al. 2019).

Relational memory ability in schizophrenia patients can be predicted from the modularity of the core hippocampal- medial temporal lobe cortical network. There is a deficit in hippocampal signaling, including increased glutamatergic signaling. Network dysconnectivity is proposed to be a major mechanism in cognitive dysfunction in schizophrenia (Avery et al. 2018).

A decrease in GM volume exists in SZ, but patients with BD showed GM volume deficits limited to the right thalamus and left insular lobe. In both disorders, WM alterations are present in the corpus callosum, superior longitudinal fasciculus, internal capsule, external capsule, posterior thalamic radiation, and fornix (Lee et al. 2020).

Working memory and particularly storage capacity is related to the posterior parietal cortex as shown by the use of the BOLD signal. Problems with working memory are one of the core symptoms of the cognitive deficits associated with schizophrenia. On the other hand, constructs like working memory are heterogenous and involve both short-term information storage, active manipulation, prioritization, and rehearsal of the stored material (Hahn et al. 2018).

Changes in GMV in the first episode of schizophrenia in patients with cognitive deficits are located by the use of VBM (Voxel based morphometric analysis). GMV is reduced in the vermis and tonsil of the cerebellum. Changes are mainly in the left supplementary motor area and bilateral precentral gyrus. Since the cerebellum is anatomically connected to the frontal and parietal cortex, it plays a very important role in both motor and cognitive tasks. So, dysfunction of the cerebellum leads to cognitive dysmetria. GMD of superior temporal gyrus is reduced (Wang et al. 2017).

Changes in GMVs occur in multiple frontal-temporal cortices in schizophrenia patients, mainly in four areas- insula, temporal cortex, llimbic system and frontal cortices. But only in patients with BD there is an association between cognitive impairment and GMV alterations (Sun et al. 2020).

Patients with schizophrenia with less cognitive intact have fewer brain structural abnormalities. There is an association between cognition and negative symptoms in schizophrenia because of common underlying substrates (Lim et al. 2021).

The use of fMRI demonstrates that most cognitive deficits are present during the first episode of the schizophrenia spectrum (Solís-Vivanco et al. 2020).

Patients with BD have a dysfunction of the dorsal and ventral systems, which are composed respectively of the prefrontal cortex, anterior cingulate cortex and the hippocampus, insula, amygdala and ventral striatum. It is not clear whether these structures are activated only during specific tasks or also at rest. Most of the studies are using BOLD signals to find which brain regions are activated during a particular task (Zovetti et al. 2020).

During reward anticipation there are significantly high levels of activation in patients with BD in particular brain regions like the dorsal anterior cingulate cortex (ACC). In patients with SZ there is a hypoactivation in the anterior insula. A negative association between SANS score and reward anticipation exists – associated BOLD response in the dorsal ACC in BD patients. Differential diagnosis can be made based on the different brain responses between BD and SZ (Smucny et al. 2021).

Patients with BD have lower grey-matter volumes in the PFC, temporal cortex, insula, and ACC. Smaller grey matter volume in the right insula can be a biomarker for BD (Wang et al. 2019).

Patients with SZ have a reduced functional connectivity in three RSNs - dorsal and ventral aspects of the medial prefrontal cortex, anterior cingulate cortex, and posterior cingulate cortex. As to MVN, LVN, and the sensorimotor network, individuals with BD show a reduced functional connectivity in only the MVN network (Jimenez et al. 2019).

From a neurobiological point of view, Schizophrenia and Bipolar Depression share common features and differ at the same time. Patients with both diagnoses have a reduced volume of the brains and high sizes of the ventricles. By using VBM (Voxel-based morphometry) many changes in brain structures are described – gray matter volume deficits in the insula, thalamus, cingulate cortex, medial frontal gyrus, middle and superior temporal gyrus in schizophrenia patients. Patients with Bipolar Depression have low levels of Gray Matter Volume (GMV) in the anterior cingulate cortex, inferior frontal gyrus, insula, middle, and superior temporal gyrus pole, and claustrum. Patients with Schizophrenia have more deficits than those with Bipolar Depression (Maggioni et al. 2017).

In Bipolar Depression and Major Depressive Disorder brain areas like the cerebellum, and particularly cerebro-cerebellar circuits are aberrant. A study of six selected seed regions in the cerebrum (He et al. 2018), reveals a weaker negative connectivity between the right subgenual anterior cingulate cortex and the cerebellar vermis and also weaker positive connectivity between the left precuneus and the left cerebellar lobule. MDD patients showed weaker positive connectivity in the left precuneus.

FA (fractional anisotropy) in white matter tracts in MDD patients is examined by using DTI (diffusion tensor imaging). Four different types of methods are used - ROI (region of interest), tract-based spatial statistics, diffusion tractography, and diffusion connectometry. It is discovered that in MDD there is a relationship between severity of depression and FA in the right medial orbitofrontal cortex, and also between age of onset of MDD and FA in the right caudal anterior cingulate cortex by using the ROI method. That relationship between FA and depression severity can be a crucial biomarker for MDD. A relationship exists between FA in the right MOFC and depression severity (Olvet et al. 2016).

ReHo, ALFF, fALFF of the brain in the resting state of depression are applied in a study (Song et al. 2020) to discover potential prodromal biomarkers for depressive disorders. Three groups of patients are included – MDD, healthy controls, and healthy controls with first-degree relatives with MDD. The regional abnormalities that were found may be associated with cognitive network disorders and emotional distress in MDD. No particular task is used, so the activity of the brain in resting state can be considered to be a state of function baseline. rfMri is used to explore the functional connection between the motor cortex, visual cortex and subcortical areas such as the hypothalamus and hippocampus (Song et al. 2020).

Many studies describe the cognitive dysfunction in patients with BD and MDD. The Wechsler scale applied to evaluate IQ and the Hamilton Depression scale to assess depression confirm cognitive deficits, especially in attention, executive functioning, verbal memory, and fluency in both disorders (Masuda et al. 2021).

Reduced fractional anisotropy is observed In MDD patients. Diffusion tensor imaging metrics extracted from regions of interest have shown reduced FA in MDD. Reduced FA in the genu of the corpus callosum, the anterior limb of the internal capsule, the cingulum bundle near the anterior cingulate cortex, and the uncinate fasciculus are present in MDD patients. A common symptom like anhedonia is negatively correlated with FA in the genu, cingulum, and uncinate fasciculus in the depressed group. Thus, anhedonia is positively correlated with reduced FA and increased radial diffusivity in white matter pathways, so the core symptom of depressive disorders is related to abnormalities in reward network connectivity.

Lots of effort is made toward the validation of biomarkers integrating neurobiological measures in network analyses. Every particular symptom in depression is associated with a particular area of the brain. Hippocampus is related to changes in appetite, sadness, loss of interest, and irritability. Another interesting brain structure, the insula was associated with loss of interest in sex and sadness, the cingulate is associated with sadness and crying, and the fusiform gyrus is associated with crying. In general, there is a connection between symptoms and brain structures (Dillon et al. 2018).

There is much evidence for the association between the thalamus, primary somatosensory cortex, and cognitive function. Also, it is known that there is a crucial relationship between these two regions and that interaction between them is very important for the cognitive process. Resting-state functional magnetic resonance imaging is used in MDD patients in search of enhanced functional connectivity between the thalamus and primary somatosensory cortex. The main symptom of MDD - anhedonia is due to an abnormal correlation between the thalamus and somatosensory prefrontal cortex (Hilland et al. 2020).

Trying to make the differential diagnosis between BD and MDD by finding neural substrates, VBM Voxel-Based Morphometry and trail-making test were used to evaluate structural and functional brain abnormalities. Patients with BD were found to have a significant main effect on diagnosis of the volumes of grey matter of the anterior cingulate cortex and left insular GM. MDD patients showed a significant inverse correlation between the left insular GM volume and TMT-A scores. In general, maybe the anterior cingulate cortex volume is a distinct endophenotype of BD. Patients with BD and MDD are exhibiting decreased insular GM volumes. It is known that the insular cortex is playing a crucial role in emotional arousal and feelings, so is assumed to be involved in a network model of higher-level cognitive control and emotional processing (Lijun et al. 2018).

The role of the amygdala is crucial in MDD. It appears that different parts of the amygdala are functionally connected to different regions contributing to the differentiation of the cerebral network mechanism of depression. Patients with MDD have hypoconnectivity between the amygdalostriatal transition area, and the basolateral, the orbitofrontal cortex, and between the ventromedial and superficial amygdala. The dysfunction of the amygdala subregional network is independent of structural changes, more interestingly hyperconnectivity and hypoconnectivity in different subregional networks may reflect imbalanced network function, which may modulate different forms of emotional and cognitive dysfunction in MDD (Matsubara et al. 2016).

In patients with MDD, a dysfunction of the thalamus and its projection cortical targets is present. There is also a reduced connectivity between prefrontal and parietal thalamus regions of interest and bilateral middle frontal gyrus and the right posterior default mode network and between the prefrontal and motor thalamus regions of interest and lateral temporal regions (Tang et al. 2019).

Discussion

Since Kraepelin's concept of dementia praecox, the primary symptom of schizophrenia is the loss of effect and volition, i.e., the disease may be identified by the presence of primary negative symptoms (Carpenter et al., 1998). Little has been phenomenologically added after Bleuler's concept of FRS and their diagnostic value, negative symptoms being a basic part of them. After the first episode of psychosis, up to 40 percent of schizophrenia patients experience persistent negative symptoms; long-term follow-up studies have not demonstrated a significant improvement in their prevalence (Eaton et al. 1995; Herbener and Harrow 2001).

Schizophrenia patients, their families, and the healthcare system all bear a heavy burden from negative symptoms, which are linked to poor functional outcomes. Negative symptoms are grouped in the avolition-apathy and expressive deficiency domains, and they may be due to other reasons or primary to schizophrenia, according to a number of studies. Research on neurobiological underpinnings and the development of cures for initial or persistent unpleasant symptoms may be hampered if this heterogeneity is not taken into consideration. The correct therapy of secondary negative symptoms that are treatable depends on improvements in negative symptom detection and routine assessment. Future research of negative symptoms should incorporate new concepts and methods of assessment if progress is to be achieved in their comprehension and treatment (Galderisi et al. 2018).

In the course of treating schizophrenia, it's crucial to gauge the severity of the negative symptoms and how they react to medications like antipsychotics. To ensure accurate results, it has been recommended that at least two distinct evaluation techniques be employed. The Positive and Negative Syndrome Scale (PANSS) was developed and standardized for typological and dimensional assessment. Other tools for measuring cognitive impairment such as SDT, Stroop test and Luria test have been developed for use as stimuli in functional MRI research.

Cognitive deficits have been found in patients with MDD and BAD as working memory impairment, with depression worsening maintenance and interference control of WM. The term pseudodementia (Kiloh 1961), may be misleading for a lot of clinicians, implementing no organic or functional changes in CNS. In fact it is a synonym for depressive cognitive impairment as a result of neurodegenerative processes in the brain. These findings have been supported by different neurocognitive tests - The Repeatable Battery for the Assessment of Neuropsychological Status (RBANS), the Wechsler Memory Scale (WMS), the clock drawing exam, and the Trail Making test.

Today the diagnosis of schizophrenia is based entirely on self-report and description of clinical symptoms. In the search of possible biomarkers fMRI is a promising method on the route towards a biologically-based diagnosis.

Up to the mid-20s, myelination and cortical alterations are consistent with normal development. The initial structural imaging finding in schizophrenia was an enlargement of the lateral ventricles. Additionally, there is a correlation between the development of negative symptoms and a loss of grey matter; this correlation is especially strong in the left temporal lobe, left cerebellum, left posterior cingulate, and left inferior parietal sulcus. The white matter anomalies most readily discernible from other locations include the cingulum bundle, left inferior and superior frontooccipital fasciculi, forceps, thalamic radiations, and left inferior and superior frontotemporal fasciculi. The discovery could be related to the fact that schizophrenia is a heterogeneous illness. In conclusion, schizophrenia disease exhibits the disconnection syndrome model and numerous inappropriate communications between various brain regions, which disturb a number of activities (Poldrack et al. 2011).

Structural brain abnormalities and negative symptoms in schizophrenia are in a close relationship. Cognitive dysfunction is evidenced by a – connectivity-cognition relationship in schizophrenia patients (Adhikari et al. 2019). Meta analytical models show an association between left MOFC thickness and negative symptoms severity (Walton et al. 2018). Patients who scored high on negative symptoms had smaller bilateral white matter volumes (Wible et al. 2001). Lower grey-matter volume in the medial prefrontal and insular cortices is present in BD and MDD with right dorsolateral prefrontal cortex, and left hippocampus, being specific to MDD (Wise et al. 2017). A lower grey-matter volume in the medial prefrontal and insular cortices is a finding in both in BD and MDD. Patients with BD have reduced volumes of hippocampal subfields, specifically in the left CA4, GCL, ML, and both sides of the hippocampal tail (Cao et al. 2017). fMRI response for many brain regions that are part of the DMN in patients with SCZ than in patients with MDD (Wang et al. 2021).

Conclusion

The spectrum of negative symptoms ranges from schizophrenia to affective disorders in terms of different extent and manifestation of cognitive-social and affective deficits. The negative symptoms in schizophrenia raise a number of research questions before neuroscience. Future research is needed to clarify the sometimes controversial findings of the brain structure and connectivity.

References

Adhikari, B. M., L. E. Hong, H. Sampath, J. Chiappelli, N. Jahanshad, P. M. Thompson, L. M. Rowland, V. D. Calhoun, X. Du, S. Chen, and P. Kochunov. 2019. "Functional network connectivity impairments and core cognitive deficits in schizophrenia." *Hum Brain Mapp* 40 (16): 4593-4605. https://doi.org/10.1002/hbm.24723.

An Introduction to the Life and Work of John Hughlings Jackson: Introduction. *Med Hist Suppl.* 2007;(26):3-34.

Avery, S. N., B. P. Rogers, and S. Heckers. 2018. "Hippocampal Network Modularity Is Associated With Relational Memory Dysfunction in Schizophrenia." *Biol Psychiatry Cogn Neurosci Neuroimaging* 3 (5): 423-432. https://doi.org/10.1016/j.bpsc.2018.02.001.

Avram, M., F. Brandl, J. Bäuml, and C. Sorg. 2018. "Cortico-thalamic hypo- and hyper-connectivity extend consistently to basal ganglia in schizophrenia." *Neuropsychopharmacology* 43(11):2239-2248. https://doi.org/10.1038/s41386-018-0059-z.

Baune, B. T., M. Brignone, and K. G. Larsen. 2018. "A Network Meta-Analysis Comparing Effects of Various Antidepressant Classes on the Digit Symbol Substitution Test (DSST) as a Measure of Cognitive Dysfunction in Patients with Major Depressive Disorder." *Int J Neuropsychopharmacol* 21 (2): 97-107. https://doi.org/10.1093/ijnp/pyx070.

Bleuler, M., and R. Bleuler. 1986. "Dementia praecox oder die Gruppe der Schizophrenien: Eugen Bleuler." *Br J Psychiatry* 149: 661-2. https://doi.org/10.1192/bjp.149.5.661.

Brady, R. O., Jr., I. Gonsalvez, I. Lee, D. Öngür, L. J. Seidman, J. D. Schmahmann, S. M. Eack, M. S. Keshavan, A. Pascual-Leone, and M. A. Halko. 2019. "Cerebellar-Prefrontal Network Connectivity and Negative Symptoms in Schizophrenia." *Am J Psychiatry* 176 (7): 512-520. https://doi.org/10.1176/appi.ajp.2018.18040429.

Chatterjee, I., V. Kumar, S. Sharma, D. Dhingra, B. Rana, M. Agarwal, and N. Kumar. 2019. "Identification of brain regions associated with working memory deficit in schizophrenia." *F1000Res* 8: 124. https://doi.org/10.12688/f1000research.17731.1.

Chechko, Natalia, Edna C. Cieslik, Veronika I. Müller, Thomas Nickl-Jockschat, Birgit Derntl, Lydia Kogler, André Aleman, Renaud Jardri, Iris E. Sommer, Oliver Gruber, and Simon B. Eickhoff. 2018. "Differential Resting-State Connectivity Patterns of the Right Anterior and Posterior Dorsolateral Prefrontal Cortices (DLPFC) in Schizophrenia." *Frontiers in Psychiatry* 9. https://doi.org/10.3389/fpsyt.2018.00211. https://www.frontiersin.org/articles/10.3389/fpsyt.2018.00211.

Chen, P., E. Ye, X. Jin, Y. Zhu, and L. Wang. 2019. "Association between Thalamocortical Functional Connectivity Abnormalities and Cognitive Deficits in Schizophrenia." *Sci Rep* 9 (1): 2952. https://doi.org/10.1038/s41598-019-39367-z.

Dal Santo, F., L. González-Blanco, L. García-Álvarez, L. de la Fuente-Tomás, Á Velasco, C. M. Álvarez-Vázquez, C. Martínez-Cao, P. A. Sáiz, M. P. García-Portilla, and J. Bobes. 2020. "Cognitive impairment and C-reactive protein in clinically stable schizophrenia outpatients: a focus on sex differences." *Sci Rep* 10 (1): 15963. https://doi.org/10.1038/s41598-020-73043-x.

Dillon, D. G., A. Gonenc, E. Belleau, and D. A. Pizzagalli. 2018. "Depression is associated with dimensional and categorical effects on white matter pathways." *Depress Anxiety* 35 (5): 440-447. https://doi.org/10.1002/da.22734.

Du, X., F. S. Choa, J. Chiappelli, K. M. Wisner, G. Wittenberg, B. Adhikari, H. Bruce, L. M. Rowland, P. Kochunov, and L. E. Hong. 2019. "Aberrant Middle Prefrontal-Motor Cortex Connectivity Mediates Motor Inhibitory Biomarker in Schizophrenia." *Biol Psychiatry* 85 (1): 49-59. https://doi.org/10.1016/j.biopsych.2018.06.007.

Eaton, W. W., R. Thara, B. Federman, B. Melton, and K. Y. Liang. 1995. "Structure and course of positive and negative symptoms in schizophrenia." *Arch Gen Psychiatry* 52 (2): 127-34. https://doi.org/10.1001/archpsyc.1995.03950140045005.

Forlim, Caroline Garcia, Leonie Klock, Johanna Bächle, Laura Stoll, Patrick Giemsa, Marie Fuchs, Nikola Schoofs, Christiane Montag, Jürgen Gallinat, and Simone Kühn. 2020. "Reduced Resting-State Connectivity in the Precuneus is correlated with Apathy in Patients with Schizophrenia." *Scientific Reports* 10 (1): 2616. https://doi.org/10.1038/s41598-020-59393-6. https://doi.org/10.1038/s41598-020-59393-6.

Galderisi, S., A. Mucci, R. W. Buchanan, and C. Arango. 2018. "Negative symptoms of schizophrenia: new developments and unanswered research questions." *Lancet Psychiatry* 5 (8): 664-677. https://doi.org/10.1016/s2215-0366(18)30050-6.

Giraldo-Chica, M., B. P. Rogers, S. M. Damon, B. A. Landman, and N. D. Woodward. 2018. "Prefrontal-Thalamic Anatomical Connectivity and Executive Cognitive Function in Schizophrenia." *Biol Psychiatry* 83 (6): 509-517. https://doi.org/10.1016/j.biopsych.2017.09.022.

Gong, J., J. Wang, S. Qiu, P. Chen, Z. Luo, J. Wang, L. Huang, and Y. Wang. 2020. "Common and distinct patterns of intrinsic brain activity alterations in major depression and bipolar disorder: voxel-based meta-analysis." *Transl Psychiatry* 10 (1): 353. https://doi.org/10.1038/s41398-020-01036-5.

Hahn, B., B. M. Robinson, C. J. Leonard, S. J. Luck, and J. M. Gold. 2018. "Posterior Parietal Cortex Dysfunction Is Central to Working Memory Storage and Broad Cognitive Deficits in Schizophrenia." *J Neurosci* 38 (39): 8378-8387. https://doi.org/10.1523/jneurosci.0913-18.2018.

Haralanova, E., S. Haralanov, A. Beraldi, H. J. Möller, and K. Hennig-Fast. 2012. "Subjective emotional over-arousal to neutral social scenes in paranoid schizophrenia." *Eur Arch Psychiatry Clin Neurosci* 262 (1): 59-68. https://doi.org/10.1007/s00406-011-0227-1.

He, Y., Y. Wang, T. T. Chang, Y. Jia, J. Wang, S. Zhong, H. Huang, Y. Sun, F. Deng, X. Wu, C. Niu, L. Huang, G. Ma, and R. Huang. 2018. "Abnormal intrinsic cerebro-cerebellar functional connectivity in un-medicated patients with bipolar disorder and major depressive disorder." *Psychopharmacology (Berl)* 235 (11): 3187-3200. https://doi.org/10.1007/s00213-018-5021-6.

Herbener, E. S., and M. Harrow. 2001. "Longitudinal assessment of negative symptoms in schizophrenia/schizoaffective patients, other psychotic patients, and depressed patients." *Schizophr Bull* 27 (3): 527-37. https://doi.org/10.1093/oxfordjournals.schbul.a006893.

Hilland, E., N. I. Landrø, B. Kraft, C. K. Tamnes, E. I. Fried, L. A. Maglanoc, and R. Jonassen. 2020. "Exploring the links between specific depression symptoms and brain structure: A network study." *Psychiatry Clin Neurosci* 74 (3): 220-221. https://doi.org/10.1111/pcn.12969.

https://doi.org/10.1093/schbul/sbaa157. http://europepmc.org/abstract/MED/33098300. https://doi.org/10.1093/schbul/sbaa157. https://europepmc.org/articles/PMC8084446. https://europepmc.org/articles/PMC8084446?pdf=render.

Jaeger, J. 2018. "Digit Symbol Substitution Test: The Case for Sensitivity Over Specificity in Neuropsychological Testing." *J Clin Psychopharmacol* 38 (5): 513-519. https://doi.org/10.1097/jcp.0000000000000941.

Jimenez, A. M., P. Riedel, J. Lee, E. A. Reavis, and M. F. Green. 2019. "Linking resting-state networks and social cognition in schizophrenia and bipolar disorder." *Hum Brain Mapp* 40 (16): 4703-4715. https://doi.org/10.1002/hbm.24731.

Jirsaraie, Robert J., Julia M. Sheffield, and Deanna M. Barch. 2018. "Neural correlates of global and specific cognitive deficits in schizophrenia." *Schizophrenia Research* 201: 237-242. https://doi.org/https://doi.org/10.1016/j.schres.2018.06.017. https://www.sciencedirect.com/science/article/pii/S0920996418303505.

Kang, L., A. Zhang, N. Sun, P. Liu, C. Yang, G. Li, Z. Liu, Y. Wang, and K. Zhang. 2018. "Functional connectivity between the thalamus and the primary somatosensory cortex in major depressive disorder: a resting-state fMRI study." *BMC Psychiatry* 18 (1): 339. https://doi.org/10.1186/s12888-018-1913-6.

Kirschner, M., A. Schmidt, B. Hodzic-Santor, A. Burrer, A. Manoliu, Y. Zeighami, Y. Yau, N. Abbasi, A. Maatz, B. Habermeyer, A. Abivardi, M. Avram, F. Brandl, C. Sorg, P. Homan, A. Riecher-Rössler, S. Borgwardt, E. Seifritz, A. Dagher, and S. Kaiser. 2021. "Orbitofrontal-Striatal Structural Alterations Linked to Negative Symptoms at

Different Stages of the Schizophrenia Spectrum." *Schizophr Bull* 47 (3): 849-863. https://doi.org/10.1093/schbul/sbaa169.

Kochunov, P., T. R. Coyle, L. M. Rowland, N. Jahanshad, P. M. Thompson, S. Kelly, X. Du, H. Sampath, H. Bruce, J. Chiappelli, M. Ryan, F. Fisseha, A. Savransky, B. Adhikari, S. Chen, S. A. Paciga, C. D. Whelan, Z. Xie, C. L. Hyde, X. Chen, C. R. Schubert, P. O'Donnell, and L. E. Hong. 2017. "Association of White Matter With Core Cognitive Deficits in Patients With Schizophrenia." *JAMA Psychiatry* 74 (9): 958-966. https://doi.org/10.1001/jamapsychiatry.2017.2228.

Kraepelin. 1886. "Compendium der Psychiatrie. Zum Gebrauche für Studirende und Aerzte. Von Dr. Emil Kraepelin Docent an der Universität, Leipzig. Leipzig, 1883 [Compendium of Psychiatry. For use by students and doctors. from dr Emil Kraepelin Lecturer at the University of Leipzig. Leipzig, 1883]." *Journal of Mental Science* 32 (138): 254-254. https://doi.org/10.1192/bjp.32.138.254. https://www.cambridge.org/core/article/compendium-der-psychiatrie-zum-gebrauche-fur-studirende-und-aerzte-von-dr-emil-kraepelin-docent-an-der-universitat-leipzig-leipzig-1883/CE79E49E1A197B25E62EF71583FFCA1C.

Lee, D. K., H. Lee, K. Park, E. Joh, C. E. Kim, and S. Ryu. 2020. "Common gray and white matter abnormalities in schizophrenia and bipolar disorder." *PLoS One* 15 (5): e0232826. https://doi.org/10.1371/journal.pone.0232826.

Lim, Keane, Jason Smucny, Deanna M. Barch, Max Lam, Richard S. E. Keefe, and Jimmy Lee. 2021. "Cognitive Subtyping in Schizophrenia: A Latent Profile Analysis." *Schizophrenia bulletin* 47 (3): 712-721.

Ma, Q., Y. Tang, F. Wang, X. Liao, X. Jiang, S. Wei, A. Mechelli, Y. He, and M. Xia. 2020. "Transdiagnostic Dysfunctions in Brain Modules Across Patients with Schizophrenia, Bipolar Disorder, and Major Depressive Disorder: A Connectome-Based Study." *Schizophr Bull* 46 (3): 699-712. https://doi.org/10.1093/schbul/sbz111.

Madeira, N., J. V. Duarte, R. Martins, G. N. Costa, A. Macedo, and M. Castelo Branco. 2020. "Morphometry and gyrification in bipolar disorder and schizophrenia: A comparative MRI study." *Neuroimage Clin* 26: 102220. https://doi.org/10.1016/j.nicl.2020.102220.

Maggioni, E., B. Crespo-Facorro, I. Nenadic, F. Benedetti, C. Gaser, H. Sauer, R. Roiz-Santiañez, S. Poletti, V. Marinelli, M. Bellani, C. Perlini, M. Ruggeri, A. C. Altamura, V. A. Diwadkar, and P. Brambilla. 2017. "Common and distinct structural features of schizophrenia and bipolar disorder: The European Network on Psychosis, Affective disorders and Cognitive Trajectory (ENPACT) study." *PLoS One* 12 (11): e0188000. https://doi.org/10.1371/journal.pone.0188000.

Malashenkova, I. K., V. L. Ushakov, N. V. Zakharova, S. A. Krynskiy, D. P. Ogurtsov, N. A. Hailov, E. I. Chekulaeva, A. Y. Ratushnyy, S. I. Kartashov, G. P. Kostyuk, and N. A. Didkovsky. 2021. "Neuro-Immune Aspects of Schizophrenia with Severe Negative Symptoms: New Diagnostic Markers of Disease Phenotype." *Sovrem Tekhnologii Med* 13 (6): 24-33. https://doi.org/10.17691/stm2021.13.6.03.

Masuda, Y., G. Okada, M. Takamura, C. Shibasaki, A. Yoshino, S. Yokoyama, N. Ichikawa, S. Okuhata, T. Kobayashi, S. Yamawaki, and Y. Okamoto. 2021. "Age-related white matter changes revealed by a whole-brain fiber-tracking method in bipolar disorder compared to major depressive disorder and healthy controls." *Psychiatry Clin Neurosci* 75 (2): 46-56. https://doi.org/10.1111/pcn.13166.

Matsubara, T., K. Matsuo, K. Harada, M. Nakano, M. Nakashima, T. Watanuki, K. Egashira, M. Furukawa, N. Matsunaga, and Y. Watanabe. 2016. "Distinct and Shared Endophenotypes of Neural Substrates in Bipolar and Major Depressive Disorders." *PLoS One* 11 (12): e0168493. https://doi.org/10.1371/journal.pone.0168493.

Olvet, D. M., L. Delaparte, F. C. Yeh, C. DeLorenzo, P. J. McGrath, M. M. Weissman, P. Adams, M. Fava, T. Deckersbach, M. G. McInnis, T. J. Carmody, C. M. Cooper, B. T. Kurian, H. Lu, M. S. Toups, M. H. Trivedi, and R. V. Parsey. 2016. "A Comprehensive Examination of White Matter Tracts and Connectometry in Major Depressive Disorder." *Depress Anxiety* 33 (1): 56-65. https://doi.org/10.1002/da.22 445.

Peterman, J. S., E. Bekele, D. Bian, N. Sarkar, and S. Park. 2015. "Complexities of emotional responses to social and non-social affective stimuli in schizophrenia." *Front Psychol* 6: 320. https://doi.org/10.3389/fpsyg.2015.00320.

Poldrack R, Mumford J., Nichols T. 2011. *Handbook of Functional MRI Data Analysis*. Cambridge University Press.

Scarpina, F., and S. Tagini. 2017. "The Stroop Color and Word Test." *Front Psychol* 8: 557. https://doi.org/10.3389/fpsyg.2017.00557.

Schneider, Kurt. 1959. *Clinical Psychopathology*. New York: Grune & Stratton.

Sekhon, Sandeep, and Raman Marwaha. 2021. *Depressive Cognitive Disorders*. StatPearls Publishing, Treasure Island (FL).

Shukla, D. K., J. J. Chiappelli, H. Sampath, P. Kochunov, S. M. Hare, K. Wisner, L. M. Rowland, and L. E. Hong. 2019. "Aberrant Frontostriatal Connectivity in Negative Symptoms of Schizophrenia." *Schizophr Bull* 45 (5): 1051-1059. https://doi.org/10. 1093/schbul/sby165.

Silberstein, J., and P. D. Harvey. 2019. "Cognition, social cognition, and Self-assessment in schizophrenia: prediction of different elements of everyday functional outcomes." *CNS Spectr* 24 (1): 88-93. https://doi.org/10.1017/s1092852918001414.

Singh, S., S. Khushu, P. Kumar, S. Goyal, T. Bhatia, and S. N. Deshpande. 2018. "Evidence for regional hippocampal damage in patients with schizophrenia." *Neuroradiology* 60 (2): 199-205. https://doi.org/10.1007/s00234-017-1954-4.

Smucny, J., L. M. Tully, A. M. Howell, T. A. Lesh, S. L. Johnson, R. C. O'Reilly, M. J. Minzenberg, S. Ursu, J. H. Yoon, T. A. Niendam, J. D. Ragland, and C. S. Carter. 2021. "Schizophrenia and bipolar disorder are associated with opposite brain reward anticipation-associated response." *Neuropsychopharmacology* 46 (6): 1152-1160. https://doi.org/10.1038/s41386-020-00940-0.

Snowdon, J. 2011. "Pseudodementia, a term for its time: the impact of Leslie Kiloh's 1961 paper." *Australas Psychiatry* 19 (5): 391-7. https://doi.org/10.3109/10398562.2011. 610105.

Solís-Vivanco, R., F. Rangel-Hassey, P. León-Ortiz, A. Mondragón-Maya, F. Reyes-Madrigal, and C. de la Fuente-Sandoval. 2020. "Cognitive Impairment in Never-Medicated Individuals on the Schizophrenia Spectrum." *JAMA Psychiatry* 77 (5): 543-545. https://doi.org/10.1001/jamapsychiatry.2020.0001.

Song, Y., X. Shen, X. Mu, N. Mao, and B. Wang. 2020. "A study on BOLD fMRI of the brain basic activities of MDD and the first-degree relatives." *Int J Psychiatry Clin Pract* 24 (3): 236-244. https://doi.org/10.1080/13651501.2020.1744663.

Squarcina, L., M. Bellani, M. G. Rossetti, C. Perlini, G. Delvecchio, N. Dusi, M. Barillari, M. Ruggeri, C. A. Altamura, A. Bertoldo, and P. Brambilla. 2017. "Similar white matter changes in schizophrenia and bipolar disorder: A tract-based spatial statistics study." *PLoS One* 12 (6): e0178089. https://doi.org/10.1371/journal.pone.0178089.

Sun, T., P. Zhao, X. Jiang, Y. Zhou, C. Li, L. Jia, and Y. Tang. 2020. "Distinct Associations of Cognitive Impairments and Reduced Gray Matter Volumes in Remitted Patients with Schizophrenia and Bipolar Disorder." *Neural Plast* 2020: 8859388. https://doi.org/10.1155/2020/8859388.

Sun, X., J. Liu, Q. Ma, J. Duan, X. Wang, Y. Xu, Z. Xu, K. Xu, F. Wang, Y. Tang, Y. He, and M. Xia. 2021. "Disrupted Intersubject Variability Architecture in Functional Connectomes in Schizophrenia." *Schizophr Bull* 47 (3): 837-848. https://doi.org/10.1093/schbul/sbaa155.

Suttkus, S., A. Schumann, F. de la Cruz, and K. J. Bär. 2021. "Working memory in schizophrenia: The role of the locus coeruleus and its relation to functional brain networks." *Brain Behav* 11 (5): e02130. https://doi.org/10.1002/brb3.2130.

Tang, S., H. Li, L. Lu, Y. Wang, L. Zhang, X. Hu, X. Bu, X. Hu, Y. Gao, Q. Gong, and X. Huang. 2019. "Anomalous functional connectivity of amygdala subregional networks in major depressive disorder." *Depress Anxiety* 36 (8): 712-722. https://doi.org/10.1002/da.22901.

Tannous, J., H. Amaral-Silva, B. Cao, M. J. Wu, G. B. Zunta-Soares, I. Kazimi, C. Zeni, B. Mwangi, and J. C. Soares. 2018. "Hippocampal subfield volumes in children and adolescents with mood disorders." *J Psychiatr Res* 101: 57-62. https://doi.org/10.1016/j.jpsychires.2018.03.003.

Tasman, Allan, Kay, Jerald, Lieberman, Jeffrey, A., First, M. B., and Michelle B. Riba. 2015. *Psychiatry*. Fourth Edition ed. Chichester, West Sussex: John Wiley & Sons, Inc.

Trémeau, F. 2006. "A review of emotion deficits in schizophrenia." *Dialogues Clin Neurosci* 8 (1): 59-70. https://doi.org/10.31887/DCNS.2006.8.1/ftremeau.

Valaparla, Vijaya Lakshmi, Ritu Nehra, Urvakhsh Meherwan Mehta, and Sandeep Grover. 2021. "Social cognitive deficits in schizophrenia and their neurocognitive correlates across the different phases of illness." *Asian Journal of Psychiatry* 55: 102501. https://doi.org/https://doi.org/10.1016/j.ajp.2020.102501. https://www.sciencedirect.com/science/article/pii/S1876201820306146.

Walton, E., D. P. Hibar, T. G. M. van Erp, S. G. Potkin, R. Roiz-Santiañez, B. Crespo-Facorro, P. Suarez-Pinilla, N. E. M. van Haren, S. M. C. de Zwarte, R. S. Kahn, W. Cahn, N. T. Doan, K. N. Jørgensen, T. P. Gurholt, I. Agartz, O. A. Andreassen, L. T. Westlye, I. Melle, A. O. Berg, L. Morch-Johnsen, A. Færden, L. Flyckt, H. Fatouros-Bergman, E. G. Jönsson, R. Hashimoto, H. Yamamori, M. Fukunaga, N. Jahanshad, P. De Rossi, F. Piras, N. Banaj, G. Spalletta, R. E. Gur, R. C. Gur, D. H. Wolf, T. D. Satterthwaite, L. M. Beard, I. E. Sommer, S. Koops, O. Gruber, A. Richter, B. Krämer, S. Kelly, G. Donohoe, C. McDonald, D. M. Cannon, A. Corvin, M. Gill, A. Di Giorgio, A. Bertolino, S. Lawrie, T. Nickson, H. C. Whalley, E. Neilson, V. D.

Calhoun, P. M. Thompson, J. A. Turner, and S. Ehrlich. 2018. "Prefrontal cortical thinning links to negative symptoms in schizophrenia via the ENIGMA consortium." *Psychological Medicine* 48 (1): 82-94. https://doi.org/10.1017/S0033291717001283. https://www.cambridge.org/core/article/prefrontal-cortical-thinning-links-to-negative-symptoms-in-schizophrenia-via-the-enigma-consortium/B7FE158F6DEAE030607B51B586C5C553.

Wang, J., P. Kochunov, H. Sampath, K. S. Hatch, M. C. Ryan, F. Xue, J. Neda, T. Paul, B. Hahn, J. Gold, J. Waltz, L. E. Hong, and S. Chen. 2021. "White matter brain aging in relationship to schizophrenia and its cognitive deficit." *Schizophr Res* 230: 9-16. https://doi.org/10.1016/j.schres.2021.02.003.

Wang, J., L. Zhou, C. Cui, Z. Liu, and J. Lu. 2017. "Gray matter morphological anomalies in the cerebellar vermis in first-episode schizophrenia patients with cognitive deficits." *BMC Psychiatry* 17 (1): 374. https://doi.org/10.1186/s12888-017-1543-4.

Wang, X., B. Cheng, N. Roberts, S. Wang, Y. Luo, F. Tian, and S. Yue. 2021. "Shared and distinct brain fMRI response during performance of working memory tasks in adult patients with schizophrenia and major depressive disorder." *Hum Brain Mapp* 42 (16): 5458-5476. https://doi.org/10.1002/hbm.25618.

Wang, X., Q. Luo, F. Tian, B. Cheng, L. Qiu, S. Wang, M. He, H. Wang, M. Duan, and Z. Jia. 2019. "Brain grey-matter volume alteration in adult patients with bipolar disorder under different conditions: a voxel-based meta-analysis." *J Psychiatry Neurosci* 44 (2): 89-101. https://doi.org/10.1503/jpn.180002.

Wei, Yange, Miao Chang, Fay Y. Womer, Qian Zhou, Zhiyang Yin, Shengnan Wei, Yifang Zhou, Xiaowei Jiang, Xudong Yao, Jia Duan, Ke Xu, Xi-Nian Zuo, Yanqing Tang, and Fei Wang. 2018. "Local functional connectivity alterations in schizophrenia, bipolar disorder, and major depressive disorder." *Journal of Affective Disorders* 236: 266-273. https://doi.org/https://doi.org/10.1016/j.jad.2018.04.069. https://www.sciencedirect.com/science/article/pii/S0165032717326058.

Wible, C. G., J. Anderson, M. E. Shenton, A. Kricun, Y. Hirayasu, S. Tanaka, J. J. Levitt, B. F. O'Donnell, R. Kikinis, F. A. Jolesz, and R. W. McCarley. 2001. "Prefrontal cortex, negative symptoms, and schizophrenia: an MRI study." *Psychiatry Res* 108 (2): 65-78. https://doi.org/10.1016/s0925-4927(01)00109-3.

Wise, T., J. Radua, E. Via, N. Cardoner, O. Abe, T. M. Adams, F. Amico, Y. Cheng, J. H. Cole, C. de Azevedo Marques Périco, D. P. Dickstein, T. F. D. Farrow, T. Frodl, G. Wagner, I. H. Gotlib, O. Gruber, B. J. Ham, D. E. Job, M. J. Kempton, M. J. Kim, Pcmp Koolschijn, G. S. Malhi, D. Mataix-Cols, A. M. McIntosh, A. C. Nugent, J. T. O'Brien, S. Pezzoli, M. L. Phillips, P. S. Sachdev, G. Salvadore, S. Selvaraj, A. C. Stanfield, A. J. Thomas, M. J. van Tol, N. J. A. van der Wee, D. J. Veltman, A. H. Young, C. H. Fu, A. J. Cleare, and D. Arnone. 2017. "Common and distinct patterns of grey-matter volume alteration in major depression and bipolar disorder: evidence from voxel-based meta-analysis." *Mol Psychiatry* 22 (10): 1455-1463. https://doi.org/10.1038/mp.2016.72.

Wylie, K. P., J. G. Harris, D. Ghosh, A. Olincy, and J. R. Tregellas. 2019. "Association of Working Memory with Distributed Executive Control Networks in Schizophrenia." *J Neuropsychiatry Clin Neurosci* 31 (4): 368-377. https://doi.org/10.1176/appi.neuropsych.18060131.

Yang, Y., S. Liu, X. Jiang, H. Yu, S. Ding, Y. Lu, W. Li, H. Zhang, B. Liu, Y. Cui, L. Fan, T. Jiang, and L. Lv. 2019. "Common and Specific Functional Activity Features in Schizophrenia, Major Depressive Disorder, and Bipolar Disorder." *Front Psychiatry* 10: 52. https://doi.org/10.3389/fpsyt.2019.00052.

Yin, Z., M. Chang, S. Wei, X. Jiang, Y. Zhou, L. Cui, J. Lv, F. Wang, and Y. Tang. 2018. "Decreased Functional Connectivity in Insular Subregions in Depressive Episodes of Bipolar Disorder and Major Depressive Disorder." *Front Neurosci* 12: 842. https://doi.org/10.3389/fnins.2018.00842.

Yuhas, Daisy. 2013. "Throughout History, Defining Schizophrenia Has Remained a Challenge (Timeline)." *Scientific American Mind.* March.

Zheng, J., X. Wei, J. Wang, H. Lin, H. Pan, and Y. Shi. 2021. "Diagnosis of Schizophrenia Based on Deep Learning Using fMRI." *Comput Math Methods Med* 2021: 8437260. https://doi.org/10.1155/2021/8437260.

Zhuo, C., C. Wang, L. Wang, X. Guo, Q. Xu, Y. Liu, and J. Zhu. 2018. "Altered resting-state functional connectivity of the cerebellum in schizophrenia." *Brain Imaging Behav* 12 (2): 383-389. https://doi.org/10.1007/s11682-017-9704-0.

Zovetti, N., M. G. Rossetti, C. Perlini, E. Maggioni, P. Bontempi, M. Bellani, and P. Brambilla. 2020. "Default mode network activity in bipolar disorder." *Epidemiol Psychiatr Sci* 29: e166. https://doi.org/10.1017/s2045796020000803.

Biographical Sketches

Petar Popov

Affiliation: Medical University of Plovdiv; University Hospital "Sveti Georgi", Plovdiv

Education: Medical University of Plovdiv – Medical Degree

Business Address: Vasil Aprilov Bul. 15 A, 4000 Plovdiv, Bulgaria

Research and Professional Experience: Assistant professor and Doctoral student

Professional Appointments: Teaching psychiatry and medical psychology; hospital work; research in neuroimaging and negative symptoms.

Publications from the Last 3 Years: 2 articles in Bulgarian medical journals

Drozdstoy Stoyanov

Affiliation: Head of the Department of Psychiatry and Medical Psychology, Medical University Plovdiv, Bulgaria. Scientific Secretary of the Research Institute. Vice President of the Bulgarian Academy of Sciences and Arts. Visiting Fellow, University of Pittsburgh, USA

Education: Graduated with MD from the Medical University of Sofia, 2002, and PhD from the Medical University of Plovdiv, 2005. Board-certified Psychiatrist, 2007. Received a post-graduate certificate from the University of Central Lancashire, UK.

Business Address: Vasil Aprilov Bul. 15 A, 4000 Plovdiv, Bulgaria

Research and Professional Experience:
- Resident in psychiatry, Military Medical Academy (2003-2005); psychiatrist at State Psychiatric Hospital (2006-2015); consultant psychiatrist in outpatient medical center (2011-ongoing).
- Elected associate professor 2008, promoted to full professor 2014. Doctor of Sciences, 2018.
- Guest Lecturer in the Universities of Copenhagen and Basel (2015), Vienna (2017), Bergen (2018). Project partner at Collaborating Center for Values Based Practice, University of Oxford, UK. Guest Editor (since 2018) and Editorial Board member (since 2020) of Current Topics in Medicinal Chemistry; Review Editor (since 2013) and Associate Editor (since 2017) of Frontiers in Psychiatry; Executive Guest Editor, CNS & Neurological Disorders-Drug Targets (since 2020); Editorial board member, Philosophy, Psychiatry and Psychology (2021-).

Honors: International Distinguished Fellow of the American Psychiatric Association and member of the Standing committee on training, Section of Psychiatry, European Union of Medical Specialists. Bronze medal from the European Society of Person Centered Healthcare.

Publications from the Last 3 Years: Authored and co-authored 200 publications, 50 of them in the last 3 years; cited about 1800 times. H-index = 24. Ranked in top 20% of the scientists in philosophy in the world by the Stanford University World Scientist and University Rankings 2022.

Stefan Popov

Affiliation: Medical University of Plovdiv; University Hospital "Sveti Georgi", Plovdiv – Head of the Clinic of Psychiatry

Education: Medical Academy of Sofia – Medical Degree

Business Address: Vasil Aprilov Bul. 15 A, 4000 Plovdiv, Bulgaria

Research and Professional Experience: research in sexual dysfunctions and microbiome of affective and alcohol use disorders

Professional Appointments: teaching psychiatry and clinical sexology; hospital work;

Honors: Associate Professor, PhD, MHS

Publications: 50 articles in Bulgarian and foreign medical journals

Chapter 2

Propriety of Proof of Concept (PoC) Trials in Interactive Social Cognition Interventions: A Program Summary of Mentalization-Based Group Therapy - *Interactional* (MBGT-*i*)

Killorin Riddell, PhD and Monty Clouse, PhD
Trauma Intervention Specialists, USA

Abstract

Program development and evaluation of a group approach to schizophrenia is described as a PoC study of the value of an attachment framework for treatment of psychiatric inpatients. Mentalization-Based Group Therapy – *interactional* (MBGT-*i*), as presented by the authors, is built from research findings in ToM, metacognition/social cognition, MCT/SCIT, and MBT, and includes a manualized curriculum that follows a guided clinical process. Changes in patients' abilities to self-reflect, take another person's perspective, and social understanding are measured according to a non-standardized *Staff Survey*, *Bell Lysaker Emotion Recognition Test* (BLERT) and the *Hinting Task Test*. Results suggest changes in the desired direction, but are not considered valid due to limitations in the experimental rigor of the research design. Observations suggest that relational concerns of safety and engagement are primary focus for group members.

In: Understanding Psychotic Disorders
Editor: Charles L. Burgess
ISBN: 979-8-88697-336-5
© 2022 Nova Science Publishers, Inc.

Introduction

A secure attachment relationship that provides an emotional bond, safe haven, comfort and calm, is what encourages human development. It is only through interactions with the social environment (primarily the family) and having needs met, that the infant begins to feel safe and to grow. The infant mentalizes his parent's responsiveness as meaningful, and it becomes his representational world and *social understanding*.

Our human need to experience *Self* and *Other* is an inborn evolutionarily-determined, psycho-biologically-represented drive intrinsic to our development into personhood. Without the recognition, connection, and appreciation from the *Other*, what will happen to us and how do we overcome it? Development results in the increasing capacity for self-regulation and the increasing capacity for differentiated relating to others.

How to best understand schizophrenia is through the concept of *social understanding*.

A review of the literature that contributes to the rationale, development, and evaluation of a program for a group approach, as considered according to the propriety of PoC for treatment of schizophrenia, is described according to this premise.

Program Rationale

'Theory of Mind'

'Theory of mind' has been applied to the investigation of schizophrenia. 'Theory of mind' (ToM) describes the mental ability to attribute thoughts, beliefs, and intentions to people in order to explain behavior. Frith (1992) proposes a relationship between schizophrenia and a mentalizing impairment that explains some of the observed symptoms: an inability to correctly interpret and predict the mental states of other people.

According to a meta-analysis of research studies by Sprong, et al. (2007) schizophrenic patients exhibit deficits in theory of mind, as measured by poor performance on "false-belief tasks," which test the ability to understand that others can hold false beliefs about events in the world; and on "intention-inference tasks," which test the ability to infer a character's intention from reading a short story. Harrington et al. (2005) find that tasks measuring ToM (second order false-belief and deception, false-belief picture-sequencing, hinting, irony comprehension, and compliance with speech maxims) consistently discriminate between schizophrenia and nonschizophrenia patient samples.

Research (Konstantakopoulos, G. et al. - 2014) also finds that impairment in theory of mind negatively affects clinical insight, the patient's awareness of their mental illness. This is related to an inability to accurately self-represent and to take the perspective of another person. According to Konstantakopoulos, et al. (2014) "therapies that teach patients perspective-taking and self-reflection skills can improve abilities in reading social cues and taking the perspective of another person."

Metacognition

A conceptualization similar to ToM, applied to the study of schizophrenia, is "metacognition," the knowledge of one's own cognitions. Metacognition includes thinking about thinking; recognizing thoughts, feelings, intentions; and making connections between events that become integrated into complex representations (Lysaker, et al. 2014). Lysaker, et al. emphasize that a focus on just symptoms alone misses treatment opportunities for schizophrenia. Interventions targeting deficits in the metacognitive abilities that allow persons to form complex ideas about themselves and others and to use that knowledge to respond to psychosocial challenges is what is needed (p. 215).

Social Cognition

In a field related to ToM and metacognition, schizophrenia has become the focus of social cognition research. Social cognition is defined as "mental operations that underlie social interactions" (Green et al. 2008). These include one's ability to perceive others' intentions and dispositions (Brothers, 1990). According to Penn et al. (1997), social cognition is a set of cognitive processes that are related to the perception, interpretation, and understanding of social information (Penn et al. 1997). Findings of social cognition impairments in schizophrenia are supported in the literature (Salva et al. 2013).

Research on social cognition impairments in schizophrenia explore four domains: (1) emotion processing, (2) theory of mind (ToM), (3) social perception, and (4) attributional style. Combs et al. (2014) organize these domains according to descriptions and measures as follows:

Domain	Description	Measure
Emotion processing	Identification or discrimination of emotional expressions. Emotional expressions reflect positive and negative expressions; emotions may range from subtle to salient.	Face Emotion Identification Test (FEIT) Bell-Lysaker Emotion Recognition Test (BLERT) Ekman Faces
Theory of mind	Ability to represent the mental states of others or make inferences about others' intentions. This includes understanding hints, false beliefs, intentions, irony, metaphor, sarcasm, and faux pas.	Hinting Task Brüne Cartoons Test of Awareness of Social Inference (TASIT)
Social perception	Perception or scanning of social details and use of contextual cues to determine emotional states or intentions.	Profile of Nonverbal Sensitivity Social Perception Scale
Attributional style	Assigning causality to positive and negative events; may emphasize ambiguous situations.	Internal, Personal, and Situational Attributions Questionnaire (IPSAQ) Ambiguous Intentions Hostility Questionnaire (AIHQ)

A meta-analysis by Fett, et al. (2011) found that overall, social cognition is more strongly associated with community functioning than neurocognition, with the strongest associations being between theory of mind and functional outcomes.

Metacognition and social cognition describe a field of research that has led to the development of treatment approaches for schizophrenia.

Metacognitive Training (MCT) (Moritz, et al. 2013) provides a manualized group approach that trains schizophrenia-spectrum patients to improve the efficacy and quality of their thinking about interpersonal situations and beliefs. Administered in up to 16 sessions in 60 minutes or less each, MCT is segmented into the following modules:

Module 1: Attribution – Blaming and Taking Credit.
Module 2: Jumping to Conclusions I.
Module 3: Changing Beliefs.
Module 4: To Empathize I.
Module 5: Memory – Over-confidence in errors.
Module 6: To Empathize II.
Module 7: Jumping to Conclusions II.
Module 8: Mood – Negative cognitive schemata.
Additional Module I: Self-Esteem.
Additional Module II: Dealing with Prejudices (Stigma).

The MCT materials consist of easy-to-read presentation slides with didactic instruction for group discussion both in words and pictures, experiential interactions such as exercises and role-playing, and videos depicting interpersonal situations and dilemmas.

Social Cognition and Interaction Training (SCIT) (Penn, et al. 2007) is another manualized group approach that uses didactic presentations, vignettes, exercises, and brief videos, depicting situations from which characters' thinking and emotions can be inferred. Sessions occur for 60 minutes each over a period of 18 to 20 weeks.

Early research on SCIT indicates improvements in theory of mind, emotional/social processing, attributions regarding unclear situations, better management of aggressiveness and patients' sense of better social relationships (Penn, et al. 2005; Combs, et al. 2007). Six months after intervention, SCIT patients manifested improved social functioning (Combs, et al. 2009).

Social Thinking

Educational programs in *Social Thinking* (Winner 2008) are associated with positive community outcomes (Crooke, et al. 2007). Social thinking describes a developmental approach that uses cognitive behavioral strategies to teach core social thinking concepts and related social skills. It is based upon Cognitive Behavior Therapy (CBT) principles (Dobson and Dozois 2001) as follows: Cognitive activity affects behavior; Cognitive activity may be monitored and altered; Desired behavior change may be influenced through CBT. Winner's classroom curriculum for Asperger's and autistic-spectrum students offers practical training in skills of self-reflection and perspective-taking.

Mentalization

Growing evidence indicates that there are essential links between the concepts of Theory of Mind (ToM), metacognition/social cognition, and mentalization, both theoretically and empirically, in that they refer to a *social understanding* which is impaired in persons with schizophrenia and related disorders. The research supports that this capacity is etiologically founded in early attachments (Bateman, A. & Fonagy, P. 2012), and that its absence is a contributing factor to violence (Bo, S. et al. 2015).

According to Allen, et al. (2002), our ability to mentalize shows us that we are human, because unlike an object such as a rock, we have a mind that actively relates to something outside itself; a mind that can think about a rock, another mind, or even itself.

Allen, et al. (2002) define mentalization as:

> ...interpreting and responding to the behavior of oneself and others in terms of intentional mental states, such as desires, feelings, beliefs, and the like. ... Especially crucial to mentalizing is this ability to represent the same situation in multiple ways, to think of alternatives, and to adopt multiple perspectives. Mentalizing, we can imagine various ways in which others may think and feel, wondering why they do what they do, striving to make their actions intelligible. We also develop a capacity for meta- representation, being able to think about our own thoughts and feelings.

Brent, et al. (2014) suggest that there are mentalization impairments in psychosis. In genetically predisposed individuals, attachment disturbances may contribute to:

1) impaired self-other understanding (mentalization disturbances)
2) Dopamine dysregulation and heightened states of awareness resulting from chronic hypothalamic-pituitary-adrenal—axis dysfunction, combined with reduced oxytocin/ mesolimbic dopamine inhibition.

Individuals with mentalization impairments may be prone to elaborating abnormal explanations of social experience, that, in conjunction with heightened states of awareness, could constitute a psychological/neurobiological vulnerability for the eventual emergence of psychotic symptoms.

Brent posits that attachment and mental health dopamine dysfunctions make possible altered conditions as follows:

- Heightened states of awareness.
- Misinterpretations of internal and external stimuli.
- Abnormal explanations of social experience.
- Difficulty discerning others' intentions.
- Confusion about one's position in the world relative to others (making us prone to paranoid or grandiose beliefs).

- An anomalous Self experience marked by a hyper-focus on inner mental states (hyper-reflexivity).
- A loss of the sense of being the subject of one's own experience (loss of ipseity).
- Preoccupation with fantasy.
- Withdrawal of interest in self-care and relationships with others.

The *Understanding Psychosis and Schizophrenia* recovery program manual (Cooke 2000) vividly describes subjective experiences of these symptoms in patient reports.

Mentalization-Based Treatment

"The overall aim of Mentalization-Based Treatment (MBT) is to improve mentalizing in the context of attachment relationships" (Lana, et al. 2017). MBT seeks to increase the patient's capacity to mentalize self and others. The focus is on the present moment and the patient's immediate state of mind. The process begins with empathic validation of the patient's experience and careful management of the patient's arousal level.

MBT is not directly concerned with content or narrative but with helping the patient to generate multiple perspectives; to free them up from being stuck in the "reality" of only one view; and to experience an array of mental states and to be able to recognize them as such (meta-representation). *Brief Mentalization-Based Group Therapy* has been found to be feasible and beneficial in the treatment of psychosis (Lana, et al. 2015; Lana et al. 2016).

Outcome Measurement

A review of the literature suggests possible instruments for measuring *social understanding* in schizophrenia. Social cognition goals, benchmarks, and milestones as extrapolated from Winner's *Social Thinking* educational program, supported by positive community functioning outcomes, provide items for a non-standardized *Staff Questionnaire* to assess patient social functioning. The questionnaire was later found to have internal reliability, suggesting that four correlated items were measuring the same construct. (Riddell and Clouse, 2020).

Items included in the *Staff Questionnaire* are as follows:

1. Client shows interest in another person's conversation.
2. Client is able to see herself/himself from the outside, as others see client.
3. Client acknowledges thoughts and feelings as his/her own.
4. Client understands and accepts another's point of view when not agreeing with it.
5. Client is aware of self-experience that is distinct from others' experience.
6. Client expresses humor and can be playful.
7. Client is flexible in adopting different points of view.
8. Client participates in conversations that are mutual and extend beyond greetings.
9. Client is able to identify and express feelings.
10. Client is able to understand that people sometimes misunderstand one another.
11. Client conveys that he/she is agent of his/her experience rather than a sense of "it happened to me."
12. Client is able to think about his/her own feelings.
13. Client is able to solve problems.
14. Client is able to sustain interest in another's situation/joys/challenges.
15. Client is able to think about the thoughts and feelings of others.

The Hinting Task

The Hinting Task (Corcoran, R., et al. 1995) was devised to test the ability of subjects to infer the true intent of indirect speech utterances. The task comprises ten short passages presenting an interaction between two characters. Each passage ends with one of the characters dropping an obvious hint. The participant is asked what the character truly meant. An appropriate response at this stage is given a score of two points and the next story is read out loud. If the subject fails to give the correct response, then the story continues, and an even more obvious hint is included. The participant is then asked, "What is the character's intent?" If a correct response is delivered, the subject is given a score of one. If the subject fails again to infer the intended meaning of both indirect speech utterances, then a score of zero is given for that item. Total score is calculated by summing the individual item scores. Range of performance is 0-20.

Bell Lysaker Emotion Recognition Task (BLERT)
The ability to recognize social cues is a building block to inferring others' emotional states and their intentions toward you. The Bell Lysaker Emotion Recognition Task (Bell, M. et al. 1997) is an audio-visual task designed to elicit a person's ability to discriminate seven emotional states (i.e., happiness, sadness, fear, disgust, surprise, anger or no emotion) given facial, voice-tonal, and upper-body movement cues. The BLERT consists of twenty-one, 10-second vignettes (using the same male actor) containing one of three monologues involving a work-related topic.

After each vignette, the tape is paused, and the participant circles the corresponding emotional label on an answer sheet. Performance is indexed as the total number of correctly identified emotions (ranging from 0 to 21). Test scores include the total number of correct responses, the number of correct positive affect responses (happy and surprise), the number of correct negative affect responses (sadness and fear), the number of correct difficult responses and number of correct easy responses. Minimum administration time is approximately 3.5 minutes per subject.

Program Development

An objects relations theoretical orientation is the basis for program development of a group treatment approach to patients with diagnoses of schizophrenia. A review of the literature suggests opportunities for clinical work. According to research on ToM, metacognition/social cognition, and mentalization; in schizophrenia the primary experience for the individual is that of *a dislocation from being understood or understanding others.*

Instead of treating symptoms of schizophrenia (i.e., hallucinations, delusions, etc.) as an anomaly to be remedied, the authors counter this formulation by suggesting a concept of symptoms of schizophrenia as *mentalizations* that can be integrated into more robust mentalizing that is informed by *social understanding*. But as Allen et al. (2002) point out, "becoming a mentalizer requires a nurturing relational context."

Attachment is the protoplasm and the gravity of human behavior. It propels us and orients all our efforts. Earliest secure attachment experiences (usually with our parents) promote healthy mentalizing, or the ability to explore outer and inner world, mind of self and other (Allen et al. 2002). But it is not only during childhood development that we grow; we are amenable to attachment influences throughout our lives.

Studies of emotional trauma contribute to an understanding of how mentalization operations might be subject to interference by environmental influences. (Riddell and Clouse 2017). The ideal laboratory to both evaluate and treat deficits in social understanding is within a group therapy format in which patients are provided live interactions for socialization and psychoeducation. Mentalizing is intrinsic to interactions and group process therapeutic factors. It is positive attachment experiences that are curative in schizophrenia as well as in trauma (Clouse and Riddell, 1999).

In their group therapy with hospitalized and outpatient populations, the authors created psycho-educational curriculum from findings on "theory of mind," metacognition/social cognition, and mentalization for group structure, and practiced an interactive mentalizing approach with the treatment aim of improving patients' *social understanding*. The group is entitled *Mentalization-Based Group Therapy-interactional* (MBGT-*i*).

The proposed program of MBGT-*i* targets deficits in social cognition for schizophrenic patients. The goals of MBGT-*i* are to increase mentalizing behavior, the ability to self-reflect, and the ability to take another person's perspective. These prove to be capacities that increase a patient's insight into his mental illness (Konstantakopoulos, G., et al. 2014).

MBGT-*i* for patients with schizophrenia uses interpersonal experiences within the live group process to heal self and other representational disturbances. Through multi-media materials, individual self-awareness is developed, and connections between feelings, thoughts, and behaviors made. MBGT-*i* shows how social situations can be perceived differently; illustrates how active mentalizations are in interactions; and depicts how our minds work in relationships.

Group members are also encouraged to consider how mentalizations affect one's experience of anger, aggression, and ability to understand one's own and another's intentions. MBGT-*i* uses the *Mentalization-Based Group Therapy Manual* (Karterud, S. 2015) and the program training, and credentialing of Mentalization Based Therapy founders, Drs. Bateman and Fonagy (2012).

The primary method is directed by a three-fold purpose: 1) that of creating an attachment context (located in the group vision that the root of mentalization is in being understood); 2) that of encouraging mentalizing in current interactions; and 3) that of fostering hope that mentalizing skills will improve community functioning.

The psychologists providing MBGT-*i* adopt a curious "not-knowing" stance, remaining open and mutually exploratory with patients. He or she is ready to model tolerance of doubt, skepticism, and ambiguity about perceptions and attributions which are initially presented as concrete and unchanging. The focus is on the subjective experience of the patient with a reasonable, comfortable, but not intensive degree of verbalized self-reflectivity. Feelings within interpersonal situations in the here-and-now are identified and linked with thoughts and behavior, while affective over-stimulation is monitored to protect optimal emotional equilibrium, and to avoid any interruption of patients' mentalizations. At all times, the psychologist keeps in mind, *What is this experience going to be like for group members?*

In MBGT-*i* the psychologists coach patients in how to understand the contexts of their own emotions, indirect communication, and the perspectives of others in social interactions, within a group empathic attachment support system. Training of main concepts occurs by didactically introducing them and by pointing them out in group interactions. A "mentalizing stance" is the guideline for group interactions.

Group materials include PowerPoint presentations that incorporate music at the start of each session (to stimulate affective engagement), u-tube, other videos (SCIT, MCT), colorful pictures, illustrations, lessons, stories, fairy tales, exercises, and interactive discussions, collected over time in an unpublished, fully referenced and documented, 191-page *Resource Manual* for psychologists (Riddell and Clouse, 2020).

The *Resource Manual* reflects object relations treatment objectives. First, the group establishes a safe "holding environment" (Mahler, et al. 1975) and a place to grow and be nurtured. Secondly, mental experience is explored. Third and fourth objectives are to improve appreciation of *Self* and *Other*. Coping skills for self-regulation is the fifth objective. Lastly the nature of attachment and its importance in resilience is taught.

The *Resource Manual* is divided into seven sections as follows:

I. Mentalization is fundamental to group process.
II. Mentalization is an activity of the mind.
III. Mentalization requires skills in self-reflection.
IV. Mentalization involves skills in perspective-taking.

V. Mentalization includes skills for understanding mental states and their connection to behavior.
VI. Mentalization grows from attachment. It is the foundation of our mental health.
VII. Mentalization supports flexible thinking and resilience.

Section I: Mentalization Is Fundamental to Group Process

The Resource Manual begins with a discussion of what group therapy is and how it is beneficial. The group vision is established and accepted by group members: MBGT-*i*'s sole purpose is to:

> foster our mentalizing by building and maintaining a supportive and caring place and time that instigates our innate wish (as humans) to be understood and to understand one another, and to be hopeful that we can always improve our understanding. Members are taught that the root of mentalization is in being understood.

Thus, group participants are spared the burden of performance in communicating well, because their capabilities to think, feel, express, and put things together, rests upon another's understanding of them. They will not be judged. The construct that "how we act affects others," is also taught; examples of how "showing interest" creates positive feelings in others, are given.

Section II: Mentalization Is an Activity of the Mind

After establishment of a safe place in opening groups, participants are invited to imagine and be curious while looking at picture slides and scenes and asking themselves and each other "What is this or that person(s) thinking or feeling?; what are those people doing together?" Visualizations are used for building self-experiences. Mentalization is explained as a concept.

Section III: Mentalization Requires Skills in Self-Reflection

Participant are presented with a guided visualization, *House of Thoughts* (Bak, et. al. 2015), and images of emotions. They explore their individual core values, and exercise their opinions by answering questions selected out of a hat. Why emotions are important is explored. Expression of thoughts and feelings is associated with building mental strength. A process for mentalizing *Self* is presented (Linehan 1993). The importance of introspection is illustrated in the fable of *Androcles and the Lion*. Self-reflection skill sets are taught. The concept that how others treat us affects us, and how we treat others affects them, is introduced.

Section IV: Mentalization Involves Skills in Perspective-Taking

Participants view a variety of stimuli that illustrate differences in *How I See It and How You See It*. The four steps of perspective taking are introduced (Winner, M. G. 2008). Mentalizing *Other* is defined as interpreting the actions of others as meaningful on the basis of intentional mental states. Exercises in reading people (Roberts, D., et al. 2016) sequences of pictures that tell a story (Moritz and Woodward 2007), perspective taking skill sets, critical elements in perspective-taking, making sense of idioms, and the four steps of communication (Winner 2008) are presented. The importance of empathy is taught, and multimedia exhibits of compassion discussed.

Section V: Mentalization Includes Skills for Understanding Mental States and Their Connection to Behavior

Participants are reminded of the concept that emotions and moods are always present, if you are self-aware, and that these can affect social interactions and vice versa. The experience of anger, invalidating environments, triggers, antecedents, and setting events for aggression are explored. How to treat anger with mentalization is taught. The definition of coping and specific coping skills are presented.

Section VI: Mentalization Grows from Attachment. It Is the Foundation of Our Mental Health

Attachment and mental health are linked conceptually with the *Wizard of Oz* analogy: *If I only had a mind*. In the Wizard of Oz, the scarecrow is isolated in a corn field with crows picking at him. His attachments with Dorothy, Tin Man, and Cowardly Lion cure him. Participants learn that, to a degree, our early attachments form us through mentalizations that develop from them. The *Still Face Experiment* with Dr. Edward Tronick video is shown (as appropriate) to illustrate the power of attachment security. *What is crazy?* is examined. Symptoms are described from the subjective experiences of patients. The psychobiological contribution of stress is explained. Attachment support is emphasized as a requirement to manage life and symptoms.

Section VII: Mentalization Supports Flexible Thinking and Resilience

Psychosis is considered from an Adaptive Information Processing (AIP) Model as an adaptive response to derailment of the AIP, and EMDR interventions (Miller 2016) are adapted for practice. Participants are encouraged to discover the meaning in the metaphor of the psychosis and how to decode it by mentalizing. *Wizard of Oz* analogy is used to suggest that psychosis is the "man behind the curtain." A diagram for mentalizing symptoms is provided and practiced with participants. Resilience is defined, its attributes specified, and strategies for building resilience practiced.

Program Evaluation

According to *Wikipedia* "Proof of concept (POC or PoC), also known as proof of principle, is a realization of a certain method or idea in order to demonstrate its *feasibility*, or a demonstration, in principle, with the aim of verifying that some concept or theory has practical potential. A proof of concept is usually small and may or may not be complete." Feasibility refers to a study of the strengths, weaknesses, risks, resources, and prospects for success of a given project. PoC study of MBGT-*i* asserts that a further assessment of benefits of this approach is recommended.

Regarding risks, the most important principle in any new treatment endeavor is to do no harm to our patients. Patients participate in behavioral interventions during MBGT-*i* focused on developing the patient's ability to identify their own thoughts and feelings, recognize others' feelings, take on another person's perspective, and interpret more-complex social situations. In addition, group therapy stimulates highly complex emotional and interpersonal interactions, which are harnessed for patients to explore their subjective understandings of others' motives while reflecting on their own motives.

As such, patients have experiences due to MBGT-*i* with a "probability and magnitude of harm or discomfort ... not greater in and of themselves than those ordinarily encountered in daily life or during the performance of routine ... psychological examinations or tests." This is the definition of *minimal risk* according to the U.S. Health and Human Services Department's document Title 45: Public Welfare, PART 46 — PROTECTION OF HUMAN SUBJECTS, Subpart A—Basic HHS Policy for Protection of Human Research Subjects, (j).

The three fundamental ethical principles for using any human subjects for research are:

1. Respect for persons: protecting the autonomy of all people and treating them with courtesy and respect and allowing for informed consent. Researchers must be truthful and conduct no deception;
2. Beneficence: The philosophy of "Do no harm" while maximizing benefits for the research project and minimizing risks to the research subjects; and
3. Justice: ensuring reasonable, non-exploitative, and well-considered procedures are administered fairly — the fair distribution of costs and benefits to *potential* research participants — and equally.

MBGT-*i* offers providers an analysis of components of risk in intentional terms and avoids over-stimulation through formulation. Concerns are defined as relational and specified as follows:

- Identification of attachment patterns – what is activated
- Challenges that are entailed
- Beliefs about the self
- Relationship of these to specific (varying) internal states
- Historical aspects placed into context

The plan for intervening in foreseeable risks to participants in MBGT-*i* is immediate contact with appropriate clinical staff members/treatment team.

Program Design

Data from MBGT-*i* provisions were collected in two samples.

Findings from the first program implementation within a community outpatient clinic are reviewed in a previous publication (Riddell and Clouse 2020). Most notable was that patient participation was 94% in this trial.

In a second trial, volunteer inpatients with diagnoses of schizophrenia, seen in once-a-week MBGT-*i*, as approved by their treatment providers, are measured according to the *Staff Questionnaire*, *Hinting Task*, and *Bell Lysaker Emotion Recognition Test* (BLERT) at pre- and post-group intervention.

The hypothesis is that patients' ability to make inferences about others' intentions and to perceive emotional cues according to the tests administered, as well as patients' general social cognition competency, as shown by clinicians' ratings of them on the *Staff Questionnaire*, will show significant changes (improvements).

Participant Criteria:	Pre- and Post-Intervention:	
Schizophrenia-Spectrum Approved by Treatment Team Patient Consent	Clinician completes: *Staff Questionnaire*	Patient completes: BLERT *Hinting Task*

Findings were not statistically analyzed due to limitations in the research (no – random sampling, controlled conditions, inter-rating reliability study, comparison group; etc.) However, once again patient participation reached above 80%, and for some cases, improvements were seen in the desired direction.

Results for MBGT-*i* participants who completed all pre- and post-measurements follow table below.

Interpretation of program data must be considered with due caution. Outlier cases were of interest in clinical grist for the mill, and information was shared with providers as patients deemed helpful.

The second study added a Consultation Group component to the program evaluation. Clinicians who provided MBGT-*i* sessions in the inpatient setting met together separately in order to participate in peer supervision, clinician training presentations, MBT research review, program development and evaluation. The MBGT Consultation Group studied process outcomes as follows:

1. MBGT -*i* is predicted to increase participants' affective expression
2. MBGT -*i* is predicted to increase participants' mentalizing in social interactions

Assigned #	Instrument	Score Pre-Test	Score Post-Test
6	Staff Questionnaire	44	49
	BLERT	9	7
	Hinting Task	15	14
8	Staff Questionnaire	58	83
	BLERT	12	14
	Hinting Task	7	11
9	Staff Questionnaire	71	64
	BLERT	17	16
	Hinting Task	9	14
14	Staff Questionnaire	80	87
	BLERT	18	18
	Hinting Task	16	17
7	Staff Questionnaire	60	60
	BLERT	12	15
	Hinting Task	16	16
11	Staff Questionnaire	66	71
	BLERT	16	13
	Hinting Task	16	17
12	Staff Questionnaire	65	70
	BLERT	19	16
	Hinting Task	19	18
10	Staff Questionnaire	78	90
	BLERT	7	9
	Hinting Task	16	18
2	Staff Questionnaire	69	56
	BLERT	15	18
	Hinting Task	17	18
5	Staff Questionnaire	45	69
	BLERT	5	11
	Hinting Task	13	10
13	Staff Questionnaire	23	46
	BLERT	6	8
	Hinting Task	13	16
3	Staff Questionnaire	59	71
	BLERT	16	18
	Hinting Task	9	18
4	Staff Questionnaire	52	74
	BLERT	18	17
	Hinting Task	11	9
1	Staff Questionnaire	55	74
	BLERT	17	13
	Hinting Task	8	9
Total/N Average	Staff Questionnaire	58.93	68.86
	BLERT	13.36	13.79
	Hinting Task	13.21	14.64

Group observation/attendance sheets were designed according to MBGT-*i* Consultation Group recommendations and collected for each session. Observations of patient were recorded in narrative with (indications of Ability or Inability to Verbalize/Display Feelings or Discuss Relationships) Reactions to Stimuli, that are listed at the top of the note (lesson objectives) are recorded according to Didn't Understand (DU); Unsuccessful Responses (UR); Successful Responses (SR).

In addition, peer review included use of the *Mentalization-Based Group Therapy Adherence and Quality Rating Scale* (MBGT-AQRS)[1], *MBGT Clinician Guidelines*[2], and discussion of session examples of non-mentalizing (Psychic Equivalence, Pretend Mode, Teleological) verses mentalizing (Karterud 2015).

Non-mentalizing according to *Psychic Equivalence* is described as the patient's exaggeration of their internal world. Any negative feeling about self is true, no other perspective is possible. Inner experience takes over and overwhelms, terrifying. Feelings are experienced as too real (i.e., I feel bad, I am bad).

Non-mentalizing according to *Pretend Mode* is described as the patient's discussion of mental states that don't feel real. Mental state is dissociated from affect. Inner experience and outer world are detached, and there is a sense of emptiness and meaninglessness.

Non-mentalizing according to *Teleogical* is described as patient's mental states judged on outcomes in the physical world. Altering a mental state depends upon something to happen in the external world.

---

[1] Managing group boundaries; Regulating group phases; Initiating and fulfilling turn taking; Engaging group members in mentalizing external events; Identifying and mentalizing events in the group; Caring for each group member; Managing authority; Stimulating discussions about group norms; Cooperation between co-therapists; Engagement, interest, and warmth; Exploration, curiosity, and not-knowing stance; Challenging unwarranted beliefs; Regulating emotional arousal; Acknowledging good mentalization; Handling pretend mode; Handling psychic equivalence; Focus on emotions; Stop and rewind; Focus on relationship between therapists and patients.

[2] Clinician maintains authority; Attention to implicit-explicit dimension of mentalizing; Intervene when there is an opportunity for, or need for, mentalizing work; Actively promote group interaction; Principle of 'No Advice Given' – Explain carefully!; Clinician notes that a patient is unable to maintain attentional control; Identify the experience of the patient rather than the content of the problem; Actively help the patient focus on a sub-dominant theme; Keep a lid on the dominant desire by letting off momentary steam; Don't forget you have parked a patient – you may have to pause the group if the patient becomes excessively anxious.

MBGT-*i* clinical observations of phenomena of non-mentalizing in the population treated were collected in transcripts of patient verbalizations during MBGT-*i* group sessions.

MBGT-*i* process outcome findings were presented at the Mentalization-Based Treatment Practitioner Training November 9 – 10, 2019 at UCLA with Drs. Bateman & Fonagy.

The consultation group's feedback from staff and patients indicated that participants verbalized acceptance, interest, enjoyment of group while it occurred, and talked favorably about it among others afterwards.

Consultation group self-evaluation according to some of the MBGT-AQRS yielded positive findings as follows:

1. Not-knowing stance: group facilitators observed to exhibit humility, patience, actively questioning members about experiences
2. Meta-Domain: Identification of the focus for the patient & agreement between patient and clinician about the focus: clear purpose of the group – to be understood and to understand others; use of multimedia to spark interest and engage with warmth
3. Domain Session Structure

Engagement: (provided in meta-domain) *Continuity with past session*: Each session review previous session; "Any thoughts?" *Identification of priorities*: Content of session specified in curriculum *Identification of focus for mentalizing*: Group exercises, activities, interactions, discussions

4. *Items* (observed behavior of provider): Encourage self-expression; Link patients together; Manage arousal levels; Clarify experience/rewind; Focus the topic; Link thoughts and feelings to interactions; Identify & explore affect; Use contrary moves to rebalance group discussion; Empathic validation; Recognize mentalizing; Contrast different perceptions; Link feelings to events and contexts; Explore and differentiate changing feelings in self and other; Ask for "thoughts then and now"; Explore narrative; Elaborate experience/perception (situation, thoughts, feelings).

The program review also suggests that our patients participating in MBGT-*i may have taught us* that which confirms our conceptualization about what is needed: an *attachment framework-object relations developmental objectives-mentalizing informed approach*, in the treatment of schizophrenia.

Process findings suggest that an increase in participants' affective expression and an increase in participants' mentalizing in social interactions, reflect two conditions of group process.

Group observations cluster around concepts of *safety* and *engagement*. According to patient verbalizations their primary needs are expressed in concerns as follows:

Group Observations:

1. Evoking mentalization depends upon a sense of safety in the group.

"What about when others are trying to trick you with their faces?"
"It can be fatal to not be read accurately if you're black and the police don't understand you."
"I may not want to show others my feelings – may not be safe."
"I may want to keep a good thing to myself."
"You may not want to show your emotions [with your facial expression]."
"To put myself into somebody else's shoes, I could catch the problems they have, and people here have a lot of problems."
"Some people may not want to show their anger."
"This isn't like prison. There aren't the prison politics here; you can be around any other [patients] that you want to, and talk with anyone you'd like to." (a few minutes later) "A person can change, if he wants to change."

2. Engagement is the most critical provision in establishing the group.

"I had a childhood without anybody helping me to understand other people"
"The desperado is like me. I'm all alone; sometimes I feel like I'm the only person in the world.
I have some people, but not close to here. It would be nice to have somebody to be with."
"I keep wishing I could meet somebody here, a patient or a staff member, who really knows a lot about alchemy, the main thing I'm most interested in, who could teach me and support my learning more about it."
"I've been thinking about forgiveness, and how big that is, hoping I can completely forgive wrong things that have been done to me, and that other people can completely forgive me."
"The character I'm like depends on the situation; sometimes I'm more like Blaming Bill [externalized anger] but this morning since I got a package, I'm like Easy Eddie [happiness]."

"At my job my boss is always joking and I don't get his jokes and I wonder if he's making fun of me, so I feel like a MY-Fault Mary character [fearful and/or sad]."

"I'm like an Easy Eddie and like to be around others who are like that too.... and *you* (referencing Facilitator) are like that too, when I see you on the unit and when I hear you from my room how you are in Aggression Reduction group."

3. A surprisingly detailed, nuanced, complete mentalization

Group member, confronted by a Parole Agent for coming late to his appointments, said he'd felt angry, unfairly picked on by her, mistreated because *"other guys weren't even coming to their appointments,"* and *"the bus I came on that day had an accident with a pedestrian, making it late."*
Facilitator: "What is your current experience in telling about this interaction?"
Group member, with genuine feeling of gratitude and some wonder, said:

"She was exactly right, she was trying to protect me! I had been doing all kinds of craziness, like going into peoples' houses even when I thought they might be at home, all kinds of things that weren't going to end up any other way than getting arrested."

Discussion

Our patients with schizophrenia have always needed additional treatment. Even though the psychosocial recovery model, the evolution of psychopharmacological approaches, and cognitive behavior therapy have offered substantial benefits, an important aspect of our patients' suffering has not been targeted and addressed directly. That overlooked aspect is our patients' difficulty with social relationships, from the point of earliest attachments, leading up to contemporary interactions with peers and staff members. Our patients have struggled with making sense of, and responding competently to, interpersonal situations. This is because they are unable to recognize their own thoughts and feelings, to fluently perceive another person's perspective, and to develop *social understanding*.

It is clear from the psychology literature that social understanding is much more complex than intelligence, neurocognition, or symptom remission. It is imperative for our work that we assist our patients in seeing through the array of indirect communications so that they "get" what's going on around them.

And, it is critical for our patients' community functioning that they develop the capacity for healthy mentalizations. Mentalization-Based Group Therapy-*interactional* is dedicated to our patients' growth in appreciating *Self* and *Other* for the promise of social support and personal well-being.

Conclusion

Proof of concept research has initiated changes in practice that have led to new findings. Evidence-based group treatment practices that remediate social cognition deficits in the population served, reduce recidivism. Information described in treatment experiences is one avenue to stimulate more study. In addition, therapy groups that increase patient participation and which patients describe as interesting, fun, and personally beneficial are good for outcomes. It is hypothesized that participation in MBGT-*i* will lead to improvements in community functioning.

MGBT-*i* has the advantage of combining, from various sources, the technical knowledge of research in 'theory of mind'; metacognition/social cognition; *Metacognitive Training*; *Social Cognition and Interaction Training*; and *Social Thinking*; into psychoeducational materials, organized within an attachment model with object relations developmental objectives, presented to patients within a mentalizing treatment process.

This review of a treatment development at our time has value. Improving care for schizophrenia is needed. Persons afflicted with associated symptoms may benefit from attachment-driven approaches that can provide practical skills to build *social understanding* and a better quality of living.

References

Allen, J. G., & Fonagy, P. (2002). *The development of mentalizing and its role in psychopathology and psychotherapy*. (Technical Report No. 02-0048.) Topeka, KS: The Menninger Clinic, Research Department.

Bak, P.; Midgley, N.; Jin L.; Zhu, J.; Wistoft, K. & Obel, C. (2015). The Resilience Program: preliminary evaluation of a mentalization-based education program. *Frontiers in Psychology*, 6: 753.

Bateman, A. & Fonagy, P. (2012). Individual techniques of the basic model. In A. W. Bateman & P. Fonagy (Eds.), *Handbook of mentalizing in mental health practice* (pp. 67–80). Washington, DC: American Psychiatric Publishing, Inc.

Bell, M., Bryson, G., and Lysaker, P. (1997). Positive and negative affect recognition in schizophrenia: a comparison with substance abuse and normal and control subjects. *Psychiatry Research*. 73:73-82.

Bo, S; Kongerslev, M.; Dimaggio, G.; Lysaker, P.; & Abu-Akel, A. (2015). Metacognition and general functioning in patients with schizophrenia and a history of criminal behavior. *Psychiatry Research*, 225: 247-253.

Brent, B. (2009). Mentalization-Based Psychodynamic Psychotherapy for Psychosis. *Journal of Clinical Psychology In Session*. Vol 65(8), 803-814.

Brent, B., Holt, D J., Keshavan, M. S., Seidman, L. J., Fonagy P. (2014). Mentalization-based Treatment for Psychosis: Linking an Attachment-based Model to the Psychotherapy for Impaired Mental State Understanding in People with Psychotic Disorders. *Israel Journal Psychiatry Related Science*. Vol 51-No 1.

Brent, B., & Fonagy, P. (2014). A mentalization-based treatment approach to disturbances of social understanding in schizophrenia. In *Social Cognition and Metacognition in Schizophrenia*. Psychopathology and Treatment Approaches. Chapter 15. pp: 245-259. Academic Press.

Brothers, L. (1990). The social brain: A project for integrating primate behavior and neurophysiology in a new domain. *Concepts in Neuroscience*, *1*, 27–61.

Clouse, M. & Riddell, K. (1999). Corporate Response to Disasters and Other Traumas, *International Journal of Emergency Mental Health,* 2, 115-125.

Combs D. R., Adams SD, Penn DL, Roberts D, Tiegreen J, Stem P. (2007). Social Cognition and Interaction Training (SCIT) for inpatients with schizophrenia spectrum disorders: preliminary findings. *Schizophrenia Research*. 91:112–6.

Combs D. R., Elerson K., Penn D. L., Tiegreen J. A., Nelson A., Ledet S. N., et al. (2009). Stability and generalization of Social Cognition and Interaction Training (SCIT) for schizophrenia: six-month follow-up results. *Schizophrenia Research* (2009): 112:196–7.

Combs, D.R., Drake, E. and Basso, M. (2014) "An Overview of Social Cognitive Treatment Interventions" In Lysaker, P., Dimaggio, G. and Brüne, M. (Eds.). *Social Cognition and Metacognition in Schizophrenia*. Elsevier Inc.

Cooke, A. (Ed.). (2000). *Understanding Psychosis and Schizophrenia*. The British Psychological Society Division of Clinical Psychology & Canterbury Christ Church University.

Corcoran, R., Mercer, G. & Frith, C. (1995). Schizohrenia, symptomatology and social inference: investigating 'theory of mind' in people with schizophrenia. *Schizophrenia Research*, 17: 5-13.

Crooke, P. J., Hendrix, R. E., Rachman, J. Y., (2007). "Brief Report: Measuring the Effectiveness of Teaching Social Thinking to Children with Asperger Syndrome (AS) and High Functioning Autism (HFA)." *Journal of Autism and Developmental Disorders*, Online Publication.

Dobson, K. and Dozois, D. (2001). "Historical and philosophical bases of the cognitive-behavioral therapies." In K. Dobson, *Handbook of Cognitive Behavioral Therapies*. The Guilford Press: New York, NY.

Fett, A. K.; Viechtbauer, W.; Dominguez, M.; Penn, D.; Os, J.; & Krabbendam, L. (2011). The relationship between neurocognition and social cognition with functional outcomes in schizophrenia: A meta-analysis. *Neuroscience and Biobehavioral Reviews*, 35: 573-588.

Frith, C. D. (1992) *The Cognitive Neuropsychology of Schizophrenia*. Psychology Press.

Frith, C. D. & Corcoran, R. (1996) Exploring 'theory of mind' in people with schizophrenia. *Psychological Medicine*, 26, 521^530.

Green, M. F., Penn, D. L., Bentall, R., Carpenter, W. T., Gaebel, W., Gur, R. C., Kring, A. M., Park, S., Silverstein, S. M., & Heinssen, R. (2008). Social cognition in schizophrenia: An NIMH workshop on definitions, assessment, and research opportunities. *Schizophrenia Bulletin*, 34(6), 1211–1220.

Harrington, L.; Siegert, R., McClure, J. (2005). Theory of Mind in schizophrenia: A critical review. *Cognitive Neuropsychiatry*, 10(4): 249-286.

Karterud, S. (2015). *Mentalization-Based Group Therapy (MBT-G): A theoretical, clinical, and research manual*. Oxford University Press.

Konstantakopoulos, G.; Ploumpidis, D.; Oulis, P.; Patrikelis, P.; Nikitopoulou, S; Papadimitriou, G.; & David, A. (2014). The relationship between insight and theory of mind in schizophrenia. *Schizophrenia Research*, 152(1): 217-222.

Lana, F., Marcos, S., Molla, L., Vilar, A. P. V. (2015). Mentalization Based Group Psychotherapy for Psychosis: A Pilot Study to Assess Safety, Acceptance and Subjective Efficacy. *International Journal of Psychology and Psychoanalysis*. 1: 2-6.

Lana, F., Cruz, M. A., Marcos, S., Romero, M., Perez, V., Marti-Bonany, J. (2016). Brief Mentalization Based Group Psychotherapy for Schizophrenic Patients. A Pilot Study to Assess Subjective Efficacy. In: *Fragilidad, Adversidad y Nuevas Terapias en las Psicosis. Madrid, 1-3 december XXI Curso Anual de Esquizofrenia* [In: *Frailty, Adversity and New Therapies in Psychoses. Madrid, December 1-3 XXI Annual Course on Schizophrenia*]. AEN. The International Society for Psychological and Social Approaches to Psychosis-ISPS.

Lana, F., Africa Cruz, M., Perez, V., and Marti Bonany, J. (2017). Social Cognition Based Therapies for People with Schizophrenia: Focus on Metacognitive and MentalizationApproaches. In *Schizophrenia Treatment*. Sage Books.

Linehan, M. (1993). *Skills training manual for treating borderline personality disorder*. The Guilford Press.

Lysaker, P., Dimaggio, G., Brune, M. (2014). Social Cognition and Metacognition in Schizophrenia: Research to Date and Directions for the Future. In Lysaker, P., Dimaggio, G., Brune (Eds.). *Social Cognition and Metacognition in Schizophrenia*. Elsevier Inc.

Mahler, M., Pine, F., and Bergman, A. (1975). *The Psychological Birth of the Human Infant*. Basic Books, Inc., Publishers. New York.

Miller, P. (2016). *EMDR Therapy for Schizophrenia and Other Psychoses*. Springer Publishing Company New York.

Moritz S, Veckenstedt R, Bohn F. Complementary group Metacognitive Training (MCT) reduces delusional ideation in schizophrenia. *Schizophr Res.* 2013; 151: 61-69.

Penn, D. L., Corrigan, P. W., Bentall, R., Racenstein, J. M., & Newman, L. (1997). Social cognition in schizophrenia. *Psychological Bulletin*, *121*, 114–132.

Penn D, Roberts DL, Munt ED, Silverstein E, Jones N, Sheitman B. (2005). A pilot study of social cognition and interaction training (SCIT) for schizophrenia. *Schizophrenia Research*. 80:357–9.

Penn, D.; Roberts, M.; Combs, D.; & Sterne, A. (2007). The development of the social cognition and interaction training program for schizophrenia spectrum disorders. *Psychiatric Services*, April, 58(4).

Riddell, K. and Clouse, M. (2020). Mentalization-Based Group Therapy-*interactional* Resource Manual (unpublished manuscript). Copyright *Trauma Intervention Specialists*.

Riddell, K. and Clouse, M. (2020). Program Development Meets Theory Development: MBGT-*i* for Schizophrenia Spectrum and Other Psychotic Disorders. *Clinical Schizophrenia & Related Psychoses*. 14:2.

Riddell, K. and Clouse, M. (2017). The 'First Wave': Earliest Intervention in Peritraumatic Processes among Survivors of Catastrophic Events. *International Journal of Emergency Mental Health and Human Resilience*. Vol. 19, No. 4, pp 1-11.

Roberts, D; Penn, D. & Combs, D. (2016). *Social Cognition and Interaction Training (SCIT)*. Ed. Barlow, D. Oxford University Press.

Sprong, M., Schothorst, E. V., Hox, J., and Van Engeland, H. (2007) Theory of Mind in Schizophrenia. *British Journal of Psychiatry*. 191, 5-13.

Salva, G. N., Vella, L., Armstrong, C. C., Penn, D. L., & Twamley, E. W. (2013). Deficits in domains of social cognition in schizophrenia: A meta-analysis of the empirical evidence. *Schizophrenia Bulletin*, *39*, 979–992.

Winner, M. G. (2008). *Think Social! A Social Thinking Curriculum for School-Age Students*. Think Social Publishing, Inc. Santa Clara, CA.

Chapter 3

Psychotic Disorders and Contributing Factors in Adolescence

Carmen Cendrero-Luengo[1],
María Jiménez-Palomares[2,*],PhD,
Juan Rodríguez-Mansilla[2], PhD,
María Jesús Rodríguez-Mansilla[3],
María Trinidad Rodríguez-Domínguez[4], PhD
and Elisa María Garrido-Ardila[2], PhD

[1]Vithas Hospital,
Sevilla, Spain
[2]ADOLOR Research Group, Medical and Surgical Department,
Medicine and Health Sciences Faculty,
University of Extremadura, Badajoz, Spain
[3]Don Benito-Villanueva Hospital, Nursing Department, Don Benito,
Badajoz, Spain
[4]ROBOLAB Research Group, Medical-Surgical Therapy Department,
Nursing and Occupational Therapy Faculty,
University of Extremadura, Badajoz, Spain

Abstract

Psychotic disorders are severe mental disorders as defined by the current edition of the Diagnostic and Statistical Manual of Mental Disorders (DSM-V). They are included in the category 'Schizophrenia spectrum and other psychotic disorders'. According to the report of the European Brain Council (EBC) and the European College of Neuropsycho-

---

* Corresponding Author's Email: mariajp@unex.es.

In: Understanding Psychotic Disorders
Editor: Charles L. Burgess
ISBN: 979-8-88697-336-5
© 2022 Nova Science Publishers, Inc.

pharmacology (ECNP) in terms of prevalence, 'every year, around 38.2% of the European population suffers from a mental disorder, constituting some 164.7 million people.'

Mental illnesses develop in a continuum process, where there are different phases. In particular, psychotic disorders start with incipient psychosis. The prognosis of psychotic disorders varies in relation to the time of detection and diagnosis of symptoms. It is considered important to detect clinical manifestations early, in order to start the treatment as soon as possible, as delay in starting treatment once symptoms have developed leads to a worse prognosis.

Adolescence is a key stage for the development of different mental disorders, particularly psychotic disorders. This stage of life is accompanied by new practices that can make us more vulnerable to suffering from a psychotic disorder or, on the contrary, play a protective role in its evolution. Contributing factors are elements that collaborate in the development of psychotic disorders. In this sense, the main risk factor is age.

The World Federation for Mental Health (WFMH) has determined that at least half of all mental health disorders appear at the age of 14, with major depression, bipolar disorder and schizophrenia being the serious mental illnesses that most affect these young people. Knowing about them, detecting them and investigating them is necessary to improve the prognosis of the pathology and to be able to carry out a correct treatment approach.

Keywords: psychotic disorders, adolescence, contributing factors, treatment and prevention

Introduction to Psychotic Disorders: Concept and Development

Throughout history, multiple theories and models have been developed about the origin, evolution and treatment of psychotic disorders. To date, the cause that triggers them is unknown, which is why they are defined as syndromes rather than diseases (Chau et al., 2018). Likewise, it is necessary to know the history of the term 'psychosis' and its literary transformation in order to understand the conceptual development of psychotic disorders. The term 'psychosis' has been used with different meanings over time in the literature. In fact, in the early days, it conceptualised different natures (Torres Ruíz 2003). For example, toxic psychosis referred to severe substance-induced mental disorders, manic-depressive psychosis referred to bipolar disorders, and organic psychosis was used to refer to dementia and delirium. The term 'psychotic' has also been used for all users or patients with severe functional impairment. Currently, the term psychotic episode or psychosis is used to group different symptoms that may appear in different mental disorders such as psychotic disorders, which involve a distortion of reality (Chau et al., 2018; Torres Ruíz 2003).

Currently, the last edition of the Diagnostic and Statistical Manual of Mental Disorders (American Psychiatric Association, 2014), states that psychotic disorders are severe mental disorders. They are grouped in the category of "Schizophrenia spectrum and other psychotic disorders". That category states that psychotic disorders are schizophrenia, other psychotic disorders and schizotypal (personality) disorder. Each psychotic disorder has a diagnosis and they are distinguished mainly by their duration, but what bring them all in the same category is having abnormalities in one or more of the following five domains: delusions, hallucinations, disorganised thinking, grossly disorganised or abnormal motor behaviour and negative symptoms (American Psychiatric Association, 2014).

The development of psychotic disorders is explained through a process of continuum, where there are different phases clearly marked by different symptoms. To understand these symptoms, the literature generally establishes two categories: positive symptoms and negative symptoms. Positive symptoms are possibly the most obvious dimension, as they are used as the main criterion for the diagnosis of psychotic disorders. These symptoms cause the patient to experience situations of arousal, perceptual disturbances, delusional behaviour etc., (Azis et al., 2021). On the other hand, negative symptoms are those that indicate an impoverishment of the patient's personality, mainly in their mood, during activities of daily living and in their social relationships (Cristóbal-Narváez et al., 2020). Among the most prominent negative symptoms are the lack of interest or initiative, apathy and lack of emotional response (Cristóbal-Narváez et al., 2020).

Regarding the evolution and development of these conditions, the latest research explains that psychotic disorders begin with incipient psychosis (Chau et al., 2018; McGorry et al., 2010). The conceptualisation of incipient psychosis is a term framed within the model of the early stages of mental disorders. This model understands mental disturbance as a gradual and continuous transition, i.e., the disorder develops through different phases, where incipient psychosis refers to the early stages of psychosis (Liu et al., 2010). Due to the continuous course of psychotic disorders, the first phase that occurs is the so-called premorbid phase, where the disorder begins to germinate (Liu et al., 2010). Its manifestations are insidious and complex to detect. The next phase to develop is the prodromal phase. This is recognised by the appearance of initial symptoms, characterised by impaired emotional, cognitive, behavioural or social functioning. In this phase there is a functional impairment of the adolescent, sometimes starting before the age of 12, and it can last for a variable period of time. It is characterised by the onset of negative symptoms, the most frequent of which are: poor concentration and attention span, lack of motivation, depressed mood, unusual worries, anxiety, irritability, distrust, deterioration of academic activities, and sleep and/or appetite disturbances, among others (Liu et al., 2010). At this point, the psychotic disorder may stagnate in this prodromal phase or may continue to evolve until the onset of the disorder's symptoms (Liu et al., 2010).

If the condition continues its development (Coentre, Levy, and Figueira 2011), the person will enter the acute phase or will have the first psychotic episode. In this phase, the positive symptoms of the disorder appear and will predominate. Among them, auditory hallucinations are significant in 80% of cases and visual hallucinations in 30%. Delusions of persecution or somatic delusions are also frequent. This stage normally lasts from 1 to 6 months (Coentre, Levy, and Figueira 2011). The last period is the remission phase in which the positive symptoms stabilise and progressively disappear, while the negative symptoms become predominant again. Apathy, lack of energy and affective flattening are frequent, although, on rare occasions, positive symptoms continue to appear. Finally, there may be relapses (relapse phase) which are considered as the appearance of positive symptoms or new onset of the acute phase. Due to this, there is also a period called the residual phase. This period is established between the acute phases, with few positive symptoms and significant deterioration due to the persistence of negative symptoms (Coentre, Levy, and Figueira 2011; Liu et al., 2010).

External Contributing Factors

Adjuvant factors or risk factors are elements that contribute to the development of a psychotic disorder. Currently, the most validated model for studying and understanding the origin of psychotic disorders is based on the interaction between genetic risk factors and environmental factors (Van Os, Rutten, and Poulton 2008). Genetic factors generate in the individual an accumulation of substantial unavoidable risk or also called innate vulnerability (Zwicker, Denovan-Wright, and Uher 2018). These factors, which are not considered sufficient for the development of a psychotic disorder, depend on their interaction with environmental factors, in this case more controllable, measurable and avoidable. Epidemiological studies have identified many environmental factors associated with an increased risk of psychosis (Zwicker, Denovan-Wright, and Uher 2018). However, no single genetic or environmental factor alone is sufficient to develop a psychotic disorder or psychosis (Zwicker, Denovan-Wright, and Uher 2018).

Age is a risk factor which is in the spotlight. The most recent literature finds that at least half of all mental health disorders appear in adolescence (Patel et al., 2021). Firstly, they identify adolescence as a vulnerable stage and a focus of risk for the development of these disorders (Patel et al., 2021). This period of the life cycle is characterised by significant changes in several domains, including brain structure and function, puberty, and social and environmental factors (Isvoranu et al., 2020; Patel et al., 2021). There are habits and routines that are acquired during adolescence that can be a fundamental trigger for mental health, irreversibly affecting its development and performance, thus constituting an environmental risk factor (Tucker 2009).

Specifically, nowadays one of the most widespread universal practices among our young people which is carried out at increasingly younger ages is the early consumption of toxic substances, mainly alcohol and cannabis. Recent research highlights that alcohol and marijuana use is higher during adolescence than at any other time of life (Thompson et al., 2021; Terry-McElrath, O'Malley, and Johnston 2013). In fact, due to the widespread and worrying use of both substances, some recent lines of research focus their investigations on the consequences and impact on mental health of the simultaneous use of both intoxicants (Terry-McElrath, O'Malley, and Johnston 2013). The combination of the two proves to be a highly compromised risk factor which exponentially increases risk (Thompson et al., 2021; Terry-McElrath, O'Malley, and Johnston 2013).

Prospective epidemiological studies have consistently shown that substance use is associated with a risk of later psychotic symptoms. In fact, they show that patients with psychosis who used toxic substances in adolescence had an earlier onset of the illness than those who did not. Therefore, it could be affirmed that the consumption of these substances anticipates or triggers the acute phase debut or prodromal symptoms of these disorders (Volkow et al., 2014; Terry-McElrath, O'Malley, and Johnston 2013; Weinstein et al., 2017). Supporting these ideas, the Dunedin cohort (Caspi et al., 2020) on cannabis use shows that its use at a young age (> 18 years) poses a risk of psychosis. However, this risk quadruples among young people who start consuming at an adolescent age (≤ 15 years) (Arseneault et al., 2004; 2002).

Both substances, cannabis and alcohol, are psychoactive/depressants of the central nervous system. However, the impact they have on brain activity has not yet been clarified and detailed. Broadly speaking, the latest research on cannabis use identifies brain regions affected by cannabis use and suggests the existence of dysregulation of circuits connecting the prefrontal cortex, the hippocampus and the striatum (Henquet et al., 2006). On the other hand, it has been shown that alcohol consumption induces a loss of white matter, as well as changes in neuronal arrangement in certain areas of the brain, such as the frontal cerebral cortex, hippocampus and cerebellum (Cookey et al., 2018). In addition, both substances cause changes in the white matter of the brain (Henquet et al., 2006; Cookey et al., 2018). There is now a growing body of evidence suggesting that alterations in connectivity between different areas of the brain are responsible for clinical symptoms or cognitive impairments observed in psychotic disorders, such as schizophrenia (Cookey et al., 2018). However, the literature assessing these changes at early stages is very limited (Cookey et al., 2018; Henquet et al., 2006).

Another factor that can risk mental health is stressful situations experienced at an early age. Increasing evidence supports the link between childhood trauma and psychosis (Varese et al., 2012; Stanton et al., 2020). Indeed, as Varese et al., estimated (Varese et al., 2012) in their meta-analysis, people with schizophrenia are almost three times more likely to have experienced adverse and traumatic events in childhood than people in the general population without mental pathology. However, most studies are based on retrospective self-reports obtained after the onset of the psychotic disorder (Stanton et al., 2020). Another increasingly widespread and therefore studied situation is the role of bullying on the mental health of our young people. Studies argue that continuous exposure to the stress of bullying and/or aggression is related to the development of psychotic symptoms, although not all victims develop one of these disorders (Van Dam et al., 2012). Early stress, in an immature brain, without coping strategies such as that of an adolescent, has a more severe and irreversible effect, creating a sensitisation to later stressors in young adulthood and adulthood (Stanton et al., 2020; Van Dam et al., 2012). A preventive role is necessary and crucial in these cases, thus avoiding irreparable consequences.

Another of the most studied factors is gender. At younger ages, psychotic disorders are more prevalent in males than in females. Previous studies detail that male subjects tend to have a higher burden of negative symptoms:

disorganisation and higher substance use than female patients (Irving et al., 2021). Other schools of thought favour pre-established behavioural roles and/or endocrine and genetic factors that condition male morbidity (Petrou, Parr, and McConachie 2018). However, the available literature is controversial and research is still needed in this area (Irving et al., 2021).

The study of sleep dysfunction as a contributing causal factor in the onset of psychosis have expanded in recent years. Small studies conducted in the mid-twentieth century in isolation already reported that sleep deprivation led to experiencing some of the positive symptoms of psychotic disorders (delusions and hallucinations), with the frequency and severity of these experiences increasing with time spent awake (Reeve, Sheaves, and Freeman 2015). Other more recent studies that focus their analysis on insomnia have shown that there are signs of insomnia that predict psychotic experiences (Reeve, Sheaves, and Freeman 2015). On the other hand, the literature also supports the theory that sleep disorder symptoms such as excessive daytime sleepiness, cataplexy and excessive snoring are predictive of psychotic experiences in the adolescent population (Lee et al., 2012). However, this line of study is rather neglected as some authors claim (Lee et al., 2012). They even criticise how once psychotic disorder has developed, sleep disorders are rarely addressed directly (Reeve, Sheaves, and Freeman 2015; Lee et al., 2012).

With respect to the emerging literature, the recently passed pandemic situation of COVID-19 has made experts focus the situation on this condition and its effects on mental health. As historical epidemiological perspectives from past pandemics and recent neurobiological evidence link infections and psychosis, there are raising concerns that SARS-CoV2 will present a significant risk for the development of these disorders (Ferrando et al., 2020). It is noteworthy that although rates of psychosis apparently increased after historical pandemics, there are so far relatively limited data correlating psychosis and SARS-CoV2. In this regards, some authors consider that only time will reveal which hypothesis is truly influential (Ferrando et al., 2020; Watson et al., 2021). These hypotheses are studied under the neurobiological model that links infections and changes in brain activity at the physiological level. Other more behavioural currents, born in Wuhan, focus on the pandemic as a period of continuous stress, with the latest reports showing high levels of anxiety, stress, distress and altered consciousness in patients. These authors go so far as to report a new-onset psychosis associated with the COVID-19 pandemic (Watson et al., 2021).

As shown in the literature, the study of risk factors that compromise mental health and could be a contributor to the development of a psychotic disorder is quite widespread and controversial. Nowadays, the global cause is not clearly described, as most of the studies analyse one factor in isolation. Therefore, the global study of these disorders during adolescence is necessary, as there is considerable evidence that supports that it is a stage of the life cycle of great vulnerability.

Prevention and Treatment

Psychotic disorders have a 1.2% prevalence and therefore are among the least common disorders. However, this could be due to methodological difficulties in their assessment, detection and follow-up. Besides, they are considered to be among the conditions that generate the most dependence and functional and social disability (Fusar-Poli et al., 2020).

About 25 years ago, the study of individuals at high Clinical Risk of Psychosis (CHR-P) (Fusar-Poli et al., 2020) was initiated in Australia. The focus of the study was on the detection and follow-up of these individuals. In fact, the detection of these truly at-risk individuals may be the key step in limiting the prevalence and incidence rate. Since this paradigm originated, the literature has grown exponentially, supporting and complementing these initial ideas (Fusar-Poli et al., 2020). Indeed, the prognosis of psychotic disorders varies in relation to the time of detection and diagnosis of symptoms. That is, the early detection of clinical manifestations is considered important in order to start treatment as soon as possible, since delay in initiating treatment once symptoms have developed leads to a worse prognosis. Therefore, detecting these clinically at-risk individuals can maximise the potential benefits of early intervention in psychosis (Lamberti et al., 2020).

Currently, in most European countries, the Early Intervention in Psychosis (EIP) model is being used to treat psychotic disorders in their different phases. Although not fully and equally implemented, pharmacological and non-pharmacological treatment is established (Albert and Weibell 2019). The two pillars of pharmacological treatment focus on the choice of antipsychotic drugs and the assessment of the problem of adherence. A good choice of drug considers side effects, mechanism of action, clinical response, as well as the stage of the disorder, individual clinical characteristics and user preferences. Besides, one of the great challenges of pharmacological treatment in psychosis is to achieve a good adherence rate (Albert and Weibell 2019).Non-pharmacological interventions complement pharmacological treatment and include psychosocial interventions such as individual therapy, family therapy, social-emotional/social skills training and community education (Clark 2016). Until recently, the focus of intervention in psychotic disorders was on the residual phase, where positive symptoms and some psychosocial dynamics were stabilised. Currently, due to the prognostic findings of these disorders, treatment is being established in the prodromal phases of the disorder through early intervention programmes (Clark 2016; Albert and Weibell 2019). Therefore, new programmes focus on the treatment of the prodromal phases, where the aim is the early detection of the disorder and the establishment of the most appropriate treatment, which leads to a better prognosis as mentioned above.

In recent decades the validity and efficacy of these interventions and early detection programmes in incipient psychosis has been confirmed and they have shown to generally improve the quality of life, well-being and future of users suffering from psychotic disorders and their families. Currently, there is a development and implementation challenge in contemporary society. According to Bouras, 2017, the possibility of carrying out good prevention by developing these programmes, in order to find an early diagnosis and individualised treatment, involves a great economic cost which is an important issue nowadays (Bouras 2017). In fact, in the report published by the WHO "Investing in Public Health", it is stated that we are facing a great imbalance between the needs for care of mental disorders and the available resources. In developed countries with well-established care systems such as Spain, between 44% and 70% of people with mental disorders do not receive treatment, with this figure rising to 90% in developing countries (Fernández, Pereira, and Torres 1995; Chapman et al., 2018).

In general, the treatment of people with psychotic disorder requires the coordination of different levels of care and different interventions. They include, in addition to pharmacological treatment, rehabilitation and social support programmes that allow them to participate in the community in a more independent and integrated way (Rocamora-Montenegro, Compañ-Gabucio, and Garcia De La Hera 2021). One of these non-pharmacological interventions is occupational therapy (OT), which can support throughout the continuum as a significant component of the treatment through purposeful and meaningful activities, influencing aspects such as autonomy in activities of daily living (ADLs), quality of life and functionality.

Over the years, the role of the occupational therapist has been established and evolved in the different phases of psychotic disorders, as has the application and establishment of this health professional in the prevention and treatment teams. As highlighted by the American Psychiatric Association,

2014, 'The essence of occupational therapy focuses on the use of activities as a means of treatment, with one goal: to improve quality of life and implement rehabilitation or habilitation for full incorporation and satisfactory development in society' (American Psychiatric Association, 2014). Years ago, the figure of the occupational therapist has been mainly present in the residual phase of the psychotic disorders. As a result, this is where the most effective treatments have been developed and implemented (Ikiugu et al., 2017). Therefore, there is a lack of awareness of its work in prevention and detection teams. In terms of treatment, from the occupational therapy approach, occupational performance is analysed, where occupational areas, skills, performance patterns, environment, activity demands and client characteristics are assessed (Ikiugu et al., 2017).

Recently, the role of the occupational therapist has been on the rise in the prodromal phases of the disorder. Their therapy approach on these phases is focused on the treatment of the affected occupational areas. Specifically, the occupational areas that tend to be affected in the prodromal phases and/or from the first psychotic episode are Instrumental Activities of Daily Living (IADL), education and/or work, leisure and free time, and social participation. In addition, performance patterns (routines, roles, habits) should also be assessed, and emphasis should be given to the family support, as users are often adolescents (Ikiugu et al., 2017). As mentioned above, adolescence is a key stage for this early detection. The habits and routines that are established at this stage of the life cycle are an essential trigger (environmental risk factors), as well as the biological predisposition (genetic factor) can be. Therefore, it is vital that a social and health professional such as the occupational therapist detects these new routines or habits in the adolescent. Apart from being immersed in a great change that makes them vulnerable, they are conditioned by socialisation agents such as family, friends and their main environments (Buchain et al., 2003). Moreover, it is at this time that they begin to acquire responsibilities, building habits, routines and roles (Buchain et al., 2003) where, as Kielhofner points out, adolescents start to become 'authors of their own lives'. The new habits are no longer mainly directed by the family, and it is common that they start to be more guided and influenced by the group of friends to which they belong. An interdisciplinary working group would comprehensively address users at high clinical risk or in the early stages of the course of the disorder. As Buchain et al., stated 'the purpose of Occupational Therapy in the early stages of these disorders is to minimise the impact of symptoms on functionality, and in the event of a psychotic break, to achieve a maximum level of functionality which is an indicator of better prognosis' (Buchain et al., 2003).

Conclusion

Delaying the start of treatment of psychotic disorders once symptoms have developed leads to a worse prognosis. Therefore, the need for the development and implementation of early detection and intervention programmes is vital. Specifically, in adolescents, this early professional detection is paramount by targeting these controllable and avoidable situations that may increase the risk of developing these irreversible disorders. All this suggests that special attention should be paid to these environmental risk factors and offer resources for their early detection in adolescence, as a key stage of the life cycle. This would lead to a better prognosis and therefore an improvement in the quality of life of these persons and their families.

References

Albert, Nikolai, and Melissa Authen Weibell. 2019. "*The Outcome of Early Intervention in First Episode Psychosis.*" Https://Doi.Org/10.1080/09540261.2019.1643703 31 (5–6): 413–24. https://doi.org/10.1080/09540261.2019.1643703.

American Psychiatric Association - APA. *Manual Diagnóstico Y Estadístico De Los Trastornos Mentales DSM-5 [Diagnostic and Statistical Manual of Mental Disorders DSM-5]*. 5a. ed. --. Madrid: Editorial Médica Panamericana, 2014.

Arseneault, Louise, Mary Cannon, Richie Poulton, Robin Murray, Avshalom Caspi, and Terrie E. Moffitt. 2002. "Cannabis Use in Adolescence and Risk for Adult Psychosis: Longitudinal Prospective Study." *BMJ (Clinical Research Ed.)* 325 (7374): 1212–13. https://doi.org/10.1136/BMJ.325.7374.1212.

Arseneault, Louise, Mary Cannon, John Witton, and Robin M. Murray. 2004. "Causal Association between Cannabis and Psychosis: Examination of the Evidence." *The British Journal of Psychiatry : The Journal of Mental Science* 184 (FEB.): 110–17. https://doi.org/10.1192/BJP.184.2.110.

Azis, Matilda, Pamela Rakhshan Rouhakhtar, Jason E. Schiffman, Lauren M. Ellman, Gregory P. Strauss, and Vijay A. Mittal. 2021. "Structure of Positive Psychotic Symptoms in Individuals at Clinical High Risk for Psychosis." *Early Intervention in Psychiatry* 15 (3): 505. https://doi.org/10.1111/EIP.12969.

Bouras, N. 2017. "Social Challenges of Contemporary Psychiatry." *Psychiatrike = Psychiatriki* 28 (3): 119–202. https://doi.org/10.22365/JPSYCH.2017.283.199.

Buchain, Patrícia Cardoso, Adriana Dias Barbosa Vizzotto, Jorge Henna Neto, and Helio Elkis. 2003. "Randomized Controlled Trial of Occupational Therapy in Patients with Treatment-Resistant Schizophrenia." *Revista Brasileira de Psiquiatria (Sao Paulo, Brazil : 1999)* 25 (1): 26–30. https://doi.org/10.1590/S1516-44462003000100006.

Caspi, Avshalom, Renate M. Houts, Antony Ambler, Andrea Danese, Maxwell L. Elliott, Ahmad Hariri, Hona Lee Harrington, Sean Hogan, Richie Poulton, Sandhya Ramrakha, Line J Hartmann Rasmussen, Aaron Reuben, Leah Richmond-Rakerd, Karen Sugden, Jasmin Wertz, Benjamin S Williams, Terrie E Moffitt, 2020. "Longitudinal Assessment of Mental Health Disorders and Comorbidities Across 4 Decades Among Participants in the Dunedin Birth Cohort Study." *JAMA Network Open* 3 (4): e203221. https://doi.org/10.1001/JAMANETWORKOPEN.2020.3221.

Chapman, Susan A., Bethany J. Phoenix, Talia E. Hahn, and Deborah C. Strod. 2018. "Utilization and Economic Contribution of Psychiatric Mental Health Nurse Practitioners in Public Behavioral Health Services." *American Journal of Preventive Medicine* 54 (6 Suppl 3): S243–49. https://doi.org/10.1016/J.AMEPRE.2018.01.045.

Chau, Hang Sze, Wai Sun Chong, Josephine Grace Wing San Wong, Gabriel Bing Kei Hung, Simon Sai Yu Lui, Sherry Kit Wa Chan, Wing Chung Chang, W. C., Hui, C. L. M., Lee, E. H. M., McGorry, P. D., Jones, P. B., & Chen, E. Y. H., 2018. "Early Intervention for Incipient Insanity: Early Notions from the 19 Th Century English Literature." *Early Intervention in Psychiatry* 12 (4): 708–14. https://doi.org/10.1111/EIP.12355.

Clark, Cameron M. 2016. "Psychosocial Treatments for Schizophrenia: An Evaluation of Theoretically Divergent Treatment Paradigms, and Their Efficacy." *Clinical Schizophrenia & Related Psychoses* 10 (1): 41–50. https://doi.org/10.3371/ CSRP.CL. 061213.

Coentre, Ricardo, Pedro Levy, and Maria Luísa Figueira. 2011. "[Early Intervention in Psychosis: First-Episode Psychosis and Critical Period]." *Acta Medica Portuguesa* 24 (1): 117–26. https://pubmed.ncbi.nlm.nih.gov/21672449/.

Cookey, Jacob, Candice E. Crocker, Denise Bernier, Aaron J. Newman, Sherry Stewart, David McAllindon, and Philip G. Tibbo. 2018. "Microstructural Findings in White Matter Associated with Cannabis and Alcohol Use in Early-Phase Psychosis: A Diffusion Tensor Imaging and Relaxometry Study." *Brain Connectivity* 8 (9): 567–76. https://doi.org/10.1089/BRAIN.2018.0611.

Cristóbal-Narváez, Paula, Tamara Sheinbaum, Araceli Rosa, Marta de Castro-Catala, Tecelli Domínguez-Martínez, Thomas R. Kwapil, and Neus Barrantes-Vidal. 2020. "Interaction of Both Positive and Negative Daily-Life Experiences with FKBP5 Haplotype on Psychosis Risk." *European Psychiatry : The Journal of the Association of European Psychiatrists* 63 (1). https://doi.org/10.1192/J.EURPSY.2019.4.

Dam, D. S. Van, E. Van Der Ven, E. Velthorst, J. P. Selten, C. Morgan, and L. De Haan. 2012. "Childhood Bullying and the Association with Psychosis in Non-Clinical and Clinical Samples: A Review and Meta-Analysis." *Psychological Medicine* 42 (12): 2463–76. https://doi.org/10.1017/S0033291712000360.

Diagnóstico, Manual, Y Estadístico, and De Trastornos Mentales. 2017. "*ACTUALIZACIÓN Suplemento Del DSM-5 ® Septiembre 2016 [DSM-5 ® Supplement UPDATE September 2016].*" http://dsm. psychiatryonline.org/.

Fernández, Juan, Joaquín Pereira, and Alberto Torres. 1995. "Una Agenda a Debate: El Informe Del Banco Mundial ' Intervenir En Salud [An Agenda for Debate: The World Bank Report ' Intervene in Health].'" *Rev Esp Salud Pública 1995;* 69 (5): 385–91.

Ferrando, Stephen J., Lidia Klepacz, Sean Lynch, Mohammad Tavakkoli, Rhea Dornbush, Reena Baharani, Yvette Smolin, and Abraham Bartell. 2020. "COVID-19 Psychosis: A Potential New Neuropsychiatric Condition Triggered by Novel Coronavirus Infection and the Inflammatory Response?" *Psychosomatics* 61 (5): 551. https://doi.org/10.1016/J.PSYM.2020.05.012.

Fusar-Poli, Paolo, Gonzalo Salazar De Pablo, Christoph U. Correll, Andreas Meyer-Lindenberg, Mark J. Millan, Stefan Borgwardt, Silvana Galderisi, S., Bechdolf, A., Pfennig, A., Kessing, L. V., van Amelsvoort, T., Nieman, D. H., Domschke, K., Krebs, M.-O., Koutsouleris, N., McGuire, P., Do, K. Q., & Arango, C., 2020. "Prevention of Psychosis: Advances in Detection, Prognosis, and Intervention." *JAMA Psychiatry* 77 (7): 755–65. https://doi.org/10.1001/JAMAPSYCHIATRY.2019.4779.

Henquet, Cécile, Araceli Rosa, Lydia Krabbendam, Sergi Papiol, Lourdes Fañanás, Marjan Drukker, Johannes G. Ramaekers, and Jim Van Os. 2006. "An Experimental Study of Catechol-O-Methyltransferase Val158Met Moderation of Δ-9-Tetrahydrocannabinol-Induced Effects on Psychosis and Cognition." *Neuropsychopharmacology* 31 (12): 2748–57. https://doi.org/10.1038/SJ.NPP.1301197.

Ikiugu, Moses N., Ranelle M. Nissen, Cali Bellar, Alexya Maassen, and Katlin Van Peursem. 2017. "Clinical Effectiveness of Occupational Therapy in Mental Health: A Meta-Analysis." *The American Journal of Occupational Therapy* 71 (5): 7105100020 p1–10. https://doi.org/10.5014/AJOT.2017.024588.

Irving, Jessica, Craig Colling, Hitesh Shetty, Megan Pritchard, Robert Stewart, Paolo Fusar-Poli, Philip McGuire, and Rashmi Patel. 2021. "Gender Differences in Clinical Presentation and Illicit Substance Use during First Episode Psychosis: A Natural Language Processing, Electronic Case Register Study," *BMJ Open* 11 (4) https://doi.org/10.1136/BMJOPEN-2020-042949.

Isvoranu, Adela Maria, Sinan Guloksuz, Sacha Epskamp, Jim Van Os, and Denny Borsboom. 2020. "Toward Incorporating Genetic Risk Scores into Symptom Networks of Psychosis." *Psychological Medicine* 50 (4): 636–43. https://doi.org/10.1017/S003329171900045X.

Lamberti, J. Steven, Viki Katsetos, David B. Jacobowitz, and Robert L. Weisman. 2020. "Psychosis, Mania and Criminal Recidivism: Associations and Implications for Prevention." *Harvard Review of Psychiatry* 28 (3): 179–202. https://doi.org/10.1097/HRP.0000000000000251.

Lee, Yu Jin, Seong Jin Cho, In Hee Cho, Joon Hwan Jang, and Seog Ju Kim. 2012. "The Relationship between Psychotic-like Experiences and Sleep Disturbances in Adolescents." *Sleep Medicine* 13 (8): 1021–27. https://doi.org/10.1016/J.SLEEP.2012.06.002.

Liu, Ping, Alexandra G. Parker, Sarah E. Hetrick, Patrick Callahan, Stefanie de Silva, and Rosemary Purcell. 2010. "An Evidence Map of Interventions across Premorbid, Ultra-High Risk and First Episode Phases of Psychosis." *Schizophrenia Research* 123 (1): 37–44. https://doi.org/10.1016/J.SCHRES.2010.05.004.

McGorry, Patrick D., Barnaby Nelson, Sherilyn Goldstone, and Alison R. Yung. 2010. "Clinical Staging: A Heuristic and Practical Strategy for New Research and Better Health and Social Outcomes for Psychotic and Related Mood Disorders." *Canadian Journal of Psychiatry. Revue Canadienne de Psychiatrie* 55 (8): 486–97. https://doi.org/10.1177/070674371005500803.

Os, Jim Van, Bart P.F. Rutten, and Richie Poulton. 2008. "Gene-Environment Interactions in Schizophrenia: Review of Epidemiological Findings and Future Directions." *Schizophrenia Bulletin* 34 (6): 1066–82. https://doi.org/10.1093/SCHBUL/SBN117.

Patel, Pooja K., Logan D. Leathem, Danielle L. Currin, and Katherine H. Karlsgodt. 2021. "Adolescent Neurodevelopment and Vulnerability to Psychosis." *Biological Psychiatry* 89 (2): 184–93. https://doi.org/10.1016/J.BIOPSYCH.2020.06.028.

Petrou, Alexandra M, Jeremy R Parr, and Helen McConachie. 2018. "Gender Differences in Parent-Reported Age at Diagnosis of Children with Autism Spectrum Disorder." *Research in Autism Spectrum Disorders* 50: 32–42. https://doi.org/http://dx.doi.org/10.1016/j.rasd.2018.02.003.

Reeve, Sarah, Bryony Sheaves, and Daniel Freeman. 2015. "The Role of Sleep Dysfunction in the Occurrence of Delusions and Hallucinations: A Systematic Review." *Clinical Psychology Review* 42 (December): 96. https://doi.org/10.1016/J.CPR.2015.09.001.

Rocamora-Montenegro, Mariá, Laura Mariá Compañ-Gabucio, and Manuela Garcia De La Hera. 2021. "Original Research: Occupational Therapy Interventions for Adults with Severe Mental Illness: A Scoping Review." *BMJ Open* 11 (10): 47467. https://doi.org/10.1136/BMJOPEN-2020-047467.

Stanton, Kate J., Brian Denietolis, Brien J. Goodwin, and Yael Dvir. 2020. "Childhood Trauma and Psychosis: An Updated Review." *Child and Adolescent Psychiatric Clinics of North America* 29 (1): 115–29. https://doi.org/10.1016/J.CHC.2019.08.004.

Terry-McElrath, Yvonne M., Patrick M. O'Malley, and Lloyd D. Johnston. 2013. "Simultaneous Alcohol and Marijuana Use among U.S. High School Seniors from 1976 to 2011: Trends, Reasons, and Situations." *Drug and Alcohol Dependence* 133 (1): 71–79. https://doi.org/10.1016/J.DRUGALCDEP.2013.05.031.

Thompson, Kara, Maria Holley, Clea Sturgess, and Bonnie Leadbeater. 2021. "Co-Use of Alcohol and Cannabis: Longitudinal Associations with Mental Health Outcomes in Young Adulthood." *International Journal of Environmental Research and Public Health 2021, Vol. 18, Page 3652* 18 (7): 3652. https://doi.org/10.3390/IJERPH18073652.

Torres Ruíz, Antonio. 2003. P. 28-30 "Revista Neurología, Neurocirugía y Psiquiatría [Neurology, Neurosurgery and Psychiatry Journal]." *Neurol Neurocir Psiquiat* 36 (1).

Tucker, Peter. 2009. "Substance Misuse and Early Psychosis." *Australasian Psychiatry: Bulletin of Royal Australian and New Zealand College of Psychiatrists* 17 (4): 291–94. https://doi.org/10.1080/10398560802657314.

Varese, Filippo, Feikje Smeets, Marjan Drukker, Ritsaert Lieverse, Tineke Lataster, Wolfgang Viechtbauer, John Read, Jim Van Os, and Richard P. Bentall. 2012. "Childhood Adversities Increase the Risk of Psychosis: A Meta-Analysis of Patient-Control, Prospective- and Cross-Sectional Cohort Studies." *Schizophrenia Bulletin* 38 (4): 661–71. https://doi.org/10.1093/SCHBUL/SBS050.

Volkow, Nora D., Gene Jack Wang, Frank Telang, Joanna S. Fowler, David Alexoff, Jean Logan, Millard Jayne, Christopher Wong, and Dardo Tomasi. 2014. "Decreased Dopamine Brain Reactivity in Marijuana Abusers Is Associated with Negative Emotionality and Addiction Severity." *Proceedings of the National Academy of Sciences of the United States of America* 111 (30). https://doi.org/10.1073/PNAS.1411228111.

Watson, Cameron J., Rhys H. Thomas, Tom Solomon, Benedict Daniel Michael, Timothy R. Nicholson, and Thomas A. Pollak. 2021. "COVID-19 and Psychosis Risk: Real or Delusional Concern?" *Neuroscience Letters* 741 (January): 135491. https://doi.org/10.1016/J.NEULET.2020.135491.

Weinstein, Aviv M., Paola Rosca, Liana Fattore, and Edythe D. London. 2017. "Synthetic Cathinone and Cannabinoid Designer Drugs Pose a Major Risk for Public Health." *Frontiers in Psychiatry* 8 (AUG): 156. https://doi.org/10.3389/FPSYT.2017.00156/BIBTEX.

Zwicker, Alyson, Eileen M. Denovan-Wright, and Rudolf Uher. 2018. "Gene-Environment Interplay in the Etiology of Psychosis." *Psychological Medicine* 48 (12): 1925–36. https://doi.org/10.1017/S003329171700383X.

Chapter 4

Narcissistic Personality Wounds in Music Therapists

**Antonia de la Torre-Rísquez[1], PhD,
Maria Isabel Ramos-Fuentes[2], PhD,
Elisa María Garrido-Ardila[3,*], PhD,
María Jiménez-Palomares[3], PhD,
Manuel Sequera-Martín[4], PhD
and Juan Rodríguez-Mansilla[3], PhD**

[1]ISOMUS, Centre of Psychology and Music Therapy,
Department of Medical-Surgical Therapy, Faculty of Medicine and Health Sciences,
University of Extremadura, Badajoz, Spain
[2]Psychiatry Area, Department of Medical-Surgical Therapy,
Faculty of Medicine and Health Sciences,
University of Extremadura, Badajoz, Spain
[3]ADOLOR Research Group, Medical and Surgical Department,
Medicine and Health Sciences Faculty,
University of Extremadura, Badajoz, Spain
[4]Centro Huella Sonora., Department of Medical-Surgical Therapy,
Faculty of Medicine and Health Sciences,
University of Extremadura, Badajoz, Spain

Abstract

Narcissism has been studied since Sigmund Freud first raised it and its interest continues to this day. Narcissistic traits will appear as a consequence of narcissistic wounds originated at an early age, during the

---

* Corresponding Author's Email: egarridoa@unex.es.

In: Understanding Psychotic Disorders
Editor: Charles L. Burgess
ISBN: 979-8-88697-336-5
© 2022 Nova Science Publishers, Inc.

maternal bond. When the individual with certain narcissistic personality traits relates to his peers, he/she projects onto them an image of himself, his traumas or his ideal. Rolando Benenzon, psychiatrist and music therapist, creator of the Benenzon Model of Music Therapy, gives special emphasis on the narcissistic wounds of the music therapist. They are a consequence of the music therapist-patient relationship and will come into play throughout the therapeutic process. They may trigger attitudes and/or actions in the music therapist in favour of him/herself and the personal needs of the music therapist, not the patient. Narcissistic wounds are activated in the music therapist when, in order to prevent the patient from leaving the therapy or the music therapist, he/she "acts out", i.e., projects his/her needs onto the patient. In view of these narcissistic wounds, the ego's defences are activated to avoid psychic pain and can form certain pathological traits that include the appearance of the well-known burnt out syndrome. Given that music therapy is becoming more relevant in the field of health sciences, the study of narcissistic wounds in music therapists is an important aspect in their training, as well as the appropriate mechanisms to prevent them from appearing, such as personal therapy and supervision of the music therapist.

Keywords: narcissism, music therapy, narcissistic wounds, narcissistic personality traits

Introduction

Music therapy is a discipline and a profession which, being transdisciplinary in nature, is difficult to define. There are different conceptions that depend on the perspective and/or culture of the group of scientists involved in its study (Wigram, Pedersen and Bonde, 2005).

From the perspective of non-verbal communication therapy, music therapy is "the technique of non-verbal communication that utilizes all the energies involved in music, opening channels of communication between the music therapist and the patient, through which the recovery process of the latter is initiated" (Benenzon, 1981). In this definition, the author covers more than just sound, music is also movement, smell, temperature, colour ... it is everything that can be perceived with the senses and sensory identity. Later, in 1998, Benenzon added to the definition that "the aim of music therapy is to improve the quality of the patient's life and to rehabilitate him/her to adapt to society" (Benenzon, 1998). In addition, it allows for the prevention, diagnosis and treatment of disorders and/or illnesses that people present (Benenzon 1998).

Similarly, the World Federation of Music Therapy defined music therapy as "the use of sound, melody, music rhythm and harmony by a professional to treat patients with problems of emotional expression, communication, mobilization and learning, which are considered important and to produce the necessary changes to achieve a better quality of life, by covering physical, emotional and cognitive needs" (Schawrcz, 2002). The latest definition of Music Therapy is from the 2011 WFMT (World Federation for Music Therapy), where it states that music therapy "is the professional use of music and its elements as an intervention in medical, educational and everyday settings with individuals, groups, families or communities seeking to optimise their quality of life and improve their physical, social, communicative, emotional, intellectual and spiritual health and well-being. Music therapy research, practice, education and clinical training are based on professional standards in accordance with cultural, social and political contexts" (World Federation of Music Therapy, 2011).

Transference, Counter transference and Acting Out

During the non-verbal communication process established in music therapy based on the perspective of the Benenzon Model, there is an exchange of reciprocal information between the music therapist and the patient called transference. This transference responds to the information that we pour into the other and that belongs to our own history, both from our non-verbal memory and from our archaic memory.

Benenzon defines transference as "placing the past in the present, in the moment of the link." (Benenzon, 2012). The patient will act and repeat behaviours from their childhood in their mother-child relationships in front of the therapist and will be able to see the therapist in the role of the father, mother, sibling and will behave in the same way as they did with their relatives at an early age. This transference will have an impact on the therapist, awakening a countertransference, that is, the feeling that emerged after the transference produced by the patient. (Benenzon, 2012).

In Music Therapy, as in any therapeutic process, the therapist-patient relationship is partial, since the therapist is the one who takes the role of helping the patient and not vice versa, however, at an unconscious level the therapeutic process can provide occasions for the therapist to satisfy his own needs, which is usually called countertransference (Bruscia, 1997).

"Countertransference is the music therapist's sense of the impact that the transference made on his unconscious." (Benenzon, 2008). In countertransference, the therapist's past experiences and the patient's transference come into play. The therapist becomes aware of the sensation of countertransference if at that very moment he or she has allowed himself or herself to return to the patient in these infantile and regressive sensations. The transference will impact on the therapist by provoking a reaction to it as a product of his countertransference (Benenzon, 2008).

The patient causes a countertransference reaction in the music therapist that makes him seek to satisfy his egotistical needs, because he feels envy due to the fact that the patient has or enjoys attention that he would like for himself. This emerges from the comparison with the other, in which the music therapist finds himself in an unfavourable situation (Amorós, Puchades, Renes and Vidal, 2018).

When a music therapist with high narcissistic personality traits feels the desire to help and believe they can help anyone, this means that the music therapist feels like they are saving their patient because they have the knowledge and ability to help them get better, but healing is between desire and hostile reality, it is achieved by the overestimation of the self and of the therapeutic probabilities. The narcissistic music therapist is willing to take risks and make decisions without being distracted by the patient's suffering and may even come to believe that it is the desire of the self to change the course of the illness. When the pathological narcissist loves himself as he would like to be loved, in that act he projects onto his admirers or possible followers, the cultivation of his admiration (De la Torre, 2022).

In the non-verbal context, during the music therapeutic process, transferential moments are appeased, which move counter-transferential events. It will be throughout the training of the music therapist during his self-experience process carried out in his specific training, when he will have to acquire and develop his own skills to safeguard and preserve himself from his own transferential moments, trying to differentiate them from the countertransferential ones in order to avoid acting out (Benenzon, 2008).

In psychoanalysis, acting out is understood as impulsive behaviour, this Anglo-Saxon term means "to carry out the act." During the therapeutic process, the music therapist is exposed to the transference of the patient, this could lead to stirring of his/her own infantile disparities, among which could be narcissistic wounds. If he/she does not become aware of it, these infantile behaviours could show themselves during therapy, which he or she is doomed to repeat, as if he/she were in the past. The probability of acting out increases in the non-verbal context (Benenzon, 2011). Bodily expression is susceptible to impulsivity since the body acts when moved by an unconscious response that has not been elaborated by the music therapist, which exposes it to acting out (Benenzon, 2011).

Narcissistic Wounds

By activating the narcissistic wounds originating in early childhood, as described above, the music therapist may lose the origin and objectives of the therapeutic process in favour of his patient and carry out different actions of his own to meet his needs or to calm unresolved conflicts (Benenzon, 2008). Psychoanalysis defines a narcissistic wound as "anything that diminishes the self-esteem of the self or diminishes the feeling of being loved by cherished objects" (Baranger, 2018).

Narcissistic wounds arise at an early age; they may originate in the intrauterine phase, at birth, postpartum or in the first and/or second year of life. They arise in the primary dual mother-baby relationship, on a biological-intuitive level, when the mother does not respond to the baby's needs, there might not be good interaction or even a lack of adequate maternal contact. This makes the baby feel helpless and a kind of emptiness, creating a basic lack of love in the child. Thus, narcissistic personality disorder could be associated with a failure in the maternal bond (Jiménez, n.d.) (Kanciper, 2010), which creates narcissistic wounds and a great vulnerability to all kinds of later traumas (Braier, 2001; Braier, 2017).

This emotional instability, which lasts a lifetime, can produce a feeling of insecurity and fragile and temporary affective relationships in the subject, as a result of a desire for union that is never satisfied. Although in his future life the individual may feel gratification in expressing his thoughts and feelings with another person, the longing to be understood without words would remain in him, similar to the basic primary (dual) relationship with the mother. This longing, originating in the irreparable loss suffered by the lack of maternal bonding, favours the feeling of loneliness (Klein, 1959). In this sense, Winnicott (1974) considers that the state of abandonment, which originates at that moment, includes moments of anguish which he calls "primitive agony" and refers to the fact that, given the baby's state of abandonment, due to failures of trust on the part of the mother or the environment, the baby was unable to integrate it as such. This state has not been provoked by the evocation of a trauma caused by an external agent, but is the result of the fact that nothing happened when it should have happened. For this reason, the individual must experience this primal agony or emptiness so that the self can then integrate it into its present experience.

Llanes (2016) points out that it is a situation that the individual has to live through in order to define a place and a desire of his own, as it is a wound that arises from the loss or abandonment of real objects, i.e., during his life, the individual will relive the wound and how he deals with it will depend on the construction of his subjectivity through the contact and links he establishes with others. In this regard, Penkin (2008) points out that: "The culmination of the constitution of the subject is going to be proposed from having lost or abandoned a number of real objects, objects and having constituted symbolic objects" (p. 295).

According to Benenzon, the narcissistic wound of the music therapist occurs when, in order to prevent the patient from abandoning him or leaving the therapy, he commits "acting out", understood as a mechanism that leads the individual to perform impulsive actions in the face of intolerable unconscious memories, that is, instead of being expressed at the level of emotions, they are manifested in the subject's behaviour, as a result of the resistance to remember (Paz, 1996). As Bruscia describes, "the music therapist meets his own needs instead of, or at the expense of, meeting the needs of the patient." The music therapist dumps his or her own unresolved conflicts on the patient and elaborates the therapeutic process based on these projections rather than on the patient's real needs (Bruscia, 1999).

The narcissistic wounds of the music therapist are activated when he feels the patient's continuity in the therapeutic process is endangered and for fear of abandoning it, he acts in a complacent way towards the patient. In the same way, these wounds are put into play in order to please and feel admired and valued by the patient in his role as "saviour" (Benenzon, 2011). (Benenzon, 2011).

In a recent research, a high level of narcissistic personality traits was found, including authority, exhibitionism and superiority. In the same study, half of the music therapists surveyed want the people closest to them, including their patients, to think they are wonderful, admire them and value them highly. They expect them to satisfy their needs and desires, showing airs and graces (De la Torre, 2022).

Supervision will be the tool adhered to the ethics of the music therapist to become aware of their narcissistic wounds, through protocols completed throughout the sessions. The figure of the supervisor should be an external agent, a spectator of the verbal account of what has happened and of the memory of what the music therapist has experienced, supported by the protocols. It is a space where traumas or anguish can be experienced, so that, when attending, they would surely experience the psychic pain of narcissistic wounds, feeling abandoned and helpless. These wounds are usually deep, therefore, many will not want to attend using any kind of excuses and in the protection of their self, they may appear overbearing or arrogant, given that their mind projects a part of the self towards objects by dividing them into good or bad and the individual tries to obsessively protect the areas they consider weak and susceptible to attack, with the consequent energy drain (Braier, 2017; Llanes, 2016; Winnicott, 1974).

In the study mentioned above, professional music therapists did not attend supervision regularly. Attending supervision could be a channel of relief, just as attending therapy on a regular basis would be, however, the results reflected that the music therapy professionals surveyed, for the most part, do not attend personal therapy on a regular basis (De la Torre, 2022).

In addition, the individual therapy of the music therapist, the care of the caregiver, will be another necessary instrument to rework the narcissistic wounds and become aware of them and to guarantee or try not to commit acting out during the therapeutic process (Benenzon, 2008).

The music therapist must always keep in mind that the patient has a body and a brain that reflects his social reality in a very particular way and any somatic alteration produces psychic reactions. In this way, when a person gets sick he will react to the pain reflecting his biopsychosocial situation, therefore, not all patients will react in the same way. Likewise, psychic alterations bring with them somatic reactions in which their emotions are expressed either externally (tremors, sweating, etc.) or internally (accelerated heart rate, modifications in the respiratory rhythm, etc.) and these can add new signs and symptoms to the condition (De la Rubia, Sancho and Cabañés, 2014). Music therapy professionals who have high or very high traits of narcissism could ignore these considerations since people with these characteristics only think about themselves, establishing a relationship with themselves in which they project their desires to be admired and loved, constantly needing the confirmation of those around them to maintain their self-esteem and do not think about the other, as a being who needs help and care, but as someone they need to be approved and admired (Benatuil, 2019).

It is very important that the music therapists with high narcissistic traits and very high personality, try to heal their wounds when they have to attend to their patients, giving more relevance to the how than to the why. (Hotchkiss, 2003).

Conclusion

In short, it is necessary to take into account this narcissistic wounds to achieve a clinical practice based on evidence and excellence, in order to ensure the best possible care for the patients or users (Sequera, 2021).

Supervision whether in individual and / or group therapy would mean that adequate self-care of the music therapist will be fundamental to offer from the viewpoint of professional ethics the highest therapeutic quality, and thus being able to emphasize aspects such as narcissistic wounds. The great difficulties for this are found in the small number of music therapists willing to take care of themselves (de la Torre, 2022) and the lack of professional regulation, which entails precarious work in the discipline (Sequera, 2021).

If we consider that music therapy is not a recognized profession in all the countries of the world and that in some countries regulation is taking years to implement whilst in others it was an arduous and expensive task despite achieving it, as in the case of Argentina, we can understand the lack of professional cohesion and an organization that ensures the health and self-care of music therapists. (Sabbatella, P and Mercadal-Brotons, M. 2014).

Another factor that influences the lack of professional adherence is found for example in countries such as Spain, where the number of existing music therapy associations exceeds twenty, granting dispersion and lack of union to the discipline. (de la Torre, 2022). Therefore, it will be necessary to become aware of the importance of self-care and personal work as a fundamental tool to achieve the highest quality in the clinical practice of the music therapist.

References

Baranger, W. (1991). El Narcisismo en Freud. En: *Estudio sobre: introducción al narcisismo de Sigmund Freud*. [In: *Study on: Sigmund Freud's introduction to narcissism*]. J. Sandler (comp.). J. Yébenes, Madrid.

Benatuil, G. O. (2019). El narcisismo y sus descontentos. Dilemas diagnósticos y estrategias de tratamiento con pacientes narcisistas [Gabbard y Crisp-Han]. *Aperturas psicoanalíticas:* [Narcissism and its discontents. Diagnostic dilemmas and treatment strategies with narcissistic patients [Gabbard and Crisp-Han]. Psychoanalytic Openings:] *Revista de psicoanálisis*, (60), 9.

Benenzon R. (2008). *La Nueva Musicoterapia*. [*The New Music Therapy*] Argentina: Lumen.

Benenzon R. (2014). *Pensando en el dolor*. [*Thinking about the pain*.] La Plata: Al Margen.

Benenzon R. (2012). *El juego del espejo y su oscuridad: la dimensión creadora*. [*The game of the mirror and its darkness: the creative dimension*] La Plata: Al Margen.

Benenzon R. (2011). *Musicoterapia de la teoría a la práctica*. [*Music therapy from theory to practice*] Madrid: Paidós.

Bleiberg, E. (1994). Normal and pathological narcissism in adolescence. *American Journal of Psychotherapy, 48*(1), 30-51.

Braier, E. (2001). Las heridas narcisistas en el trauma psíquico temprano. Teoría y clínica. [*Narcissistic wounds in early psychic trauma. Theory and clinic.*] Disponible en: https://www.raco.cat/index.php/Intercanvis/article/ view/355158.

Braier, E. (2017). Psicoanálisis y Psicoterapia psicoanalítica a la luz de una tercera tópica freudiana. [Psychoanalysis and psychoanalytic psychotherapy in the light of a third Freudian topic.] *Revista Pensamiento Psicoanalítico, 1*, 32-38.

Bruscia, K. E. (1998). *The Dynamics of Music Psychotherapy*. Gilsum (New Hampshire, USA): Barcelona Publishers.

Cohen, D. E. (2020). *Las bases neurobiológicas del trastorno límite de la perso- nalidad: Un modelo de procesamiento sistémico*. [*The neurobiological basis of borderline personality disorder: A systemic processing model*.] Editorial Autores de Argentina.

De la Rubia, J.E., Sancho, P. y Cabañés, C. (2014). Impacto fisiológico de la musicoterapia en la depresión, ansiedad, y bienestar del paciente con demencia tipo Alzheimer. Valoración de la utilización de cuestionarios para cuantificarlo. [Physiological impact of music therapy on depression, anxiety, and well-being in patients with dementia of the Alzheimer type. Assessment of the use of questionnaires to quantify it.] *European Journal of Education and Psychology, 4*(2):131-140.

De la Torre, A. (2022). *Estudio comparativo entre el síndrome fatiga de la compasión y el narcisismo en musicoterapeutas de españa*. [*Comparative study between compassion fatigue syndrome and narcissism in music therapists from Spain*.] (Doctoral dissertation, Universidad de Salamanca).

Freud, s. (1914). *Introducción del Narcisismo. Obras completas (OC)*. [*Introduction to Narcissism. Complete Works*] Vol. XIV. Bue- nos Aires: Amorrortu Editores.

Freud, S. (1914). *Recordar, repetir y elaborar. Obras completas*, [*Remember, repeat and elaborate. Complete works*] *12*, 145-157.

Freud, S. (1920). *Más allá del principio del placer* [*Beyond the Pleasure Principle*], *O. C.*, vol. XVIII. Buenos Aires: Amorrortu Editores.

Kernberg, O. (1997): *Desórdenes fronterizos y narcisismo patológico* [*Borderline disorders and pathological narcissism*] (E. Abreu, Trad.). México, Paidós. (trabajo original publicado en 1975).

Kernberg, O. (1997): *La agresión en las perversiones y en los desórdenes de la personalidad* [*Aggression in perversions and personality disorders*] (J. Piatigorski, Trad.). México: Paidós (Trabajo original publicado en 1992).

Klein M. (1959). *Sobre el sentimiento de soledad* [About the feeling of loneliness]. Buenos Aires: Hormé.

Kramer, U., Pascual-Leone, A., Rohde, K.B., Sachse, R. (2018). The role of shame and self-compassion in psychotherapy for narcissistic personality disorder. *Clinical Psychology & Psychotherapy, 25*(2), 272-282.

LLanes, J. C. (2016). Sobre la Herida Narcisista y el Trabajo de Duelo [On the Narcissistic Wound and the Work of Mourning]. *Revista Letra en Psicoanálisis*. 2(2):1-9.

Martín, M. S. (2021). *Estudio sobre la prevalencia del síndrome de burnt-out y satisfacción laboral en musicoterapeutas de españa* [Study on the prevalence of burnt-out syndrome and job satisfaction in music therapists in Spain] (Doctoral dissertation, Universidad de Salamanca).

Morrison, A. P. (2011). The psychodynamics of shame. En R. L. Dearing y J. P. Tangney (Eds.), *Shame in the therapy hour* (pp. 23-43). Washington, DC: American Psychological Association. https://doi.org/10.1037/12326-001.

Paz, C.A. (1996). "Actuación" (acting-out): 1905-1996. Orígenes, evolución y alcances actuales de esta noción freudiana [Origins, evolution and current scope of this Freudian notion]. *Revista de Psicoanálisis*. 24,167-180.

Sabbatella, P. y Mercadal-Brotons, M. (2014). Perfil profesional y laboral de los musicoterapeutas españoles: Un estudio descriptivo [Professional and labor profile of Spanish music therapists: A descriptive study]. *Revista Brasileira de Musicoterapia*, 17, 6-16.

Schawrcz, V. (2002). La musicoterapia: análisis de definiciones, caracterización de su campo de especificidad [Music therapy: analysis of definitions, characterization of its field of specificity]. *Portal de revistas científicas y arbitradas de la UNAM 3* (2), 35-52.

Sequera-Martín, M., Ramos-Fuentes, M. I., Garrido-Ardila, E. M., Sánchez-Sánchez, C., Torre-Risquez, A. D. L., & Rodríguez-Mansilla, J. (2021). Prevalence of Burnout Syndrome and Job Satisfaction in Music Therapists in Spain: A Cross-Sectional, Descriptive Study. *International journal of environmental research and public health*, 18(17), 9108.

Wigram, T., Pedersen, I. N., y Bonde, L. O. (2005). *Guía completa de musicoterapia: teoría, práctica clínica, investigación y formación* [Complete guide to music therapy: theory, clinical practice, research and training]. Vitoria- Gasteiz: AgrupArte Producciones.

Winnicott, D. (1974). Temor al derrumbe [Fear of collapse]. *Psicoan. 4* (2):269-280.

Yun, H. J., & Hyun, M. H. (2018). The Influence of Covert Narcissistic Tendency on Interpersonal Satisfaction: The Mediating Effect of Ambivalence over Emotional Expressiveness. *Korean Journal of Stress Research, 26*(4), 332-339.

Zabalza, S. (2019). El cuerpo: más allá del falo, la imagen y la castración [The body: beyond the phallus, the image and castration]. *Psicoanáli- sis En La Universidad*, (3), 113-121.

Bibliography

A clinical introduction to psychosis: foundations for clinical psychologists and neuropsychologists

LCCN	2019955909
Type of material	Book
Main title	A clinical introduction to psychosis: foundations for clinical psychologists and neuropsychologists / edited by Johanna C. Badcock, Georgie Paulik.
Published/Created	London: Academic Press, an imprint of Elsevier, [2020]
Published/Produced	©2020
Description	xix, 714 pages: illustrations; 23 cm
ISBN	9780128150122
	0128150122
LC classification	RC512 .C544 2020
Related names	Badcock, Johanna C., editor.
	Paulik, Georgie, editor.
Summary	"This practical guide outlines the latest advances in understanding and treating psychotic symptoms and disorders, articulating step-by-step the clinical skills and knowledge required to effectively treat this patient population. A Clinical Introduction to Psychosis takes an evidence-based approach that encourages a wider perspective on clinical practice, with chapters covering stigma and bias, cultural factors, the importance of social functioning, physical health, sleep, and more. A broad array of treatment modalities are discussed, including cognitive behavioral therapy, cognitive remediation, psychosocial interventions, trauma-informed therapies, and recovery-oriented practice. The book

Contents

also provides a concise overview of the latest advances regarding cognitive profiles in people with psychotic disorders, the developmental progression of cognitive abilities, and the clinical relevance of cognitive dysfunction. The book additionally familiarizes readers with issues and controversies surrounding diagnostic classification, transdiagnostic expression, and dimensional assessment of symptoms in psychosis." - Publisher's description

Section One: The basics. What is psychosis? / Clair de la Lune, Evie Glasshouse, Clara S. Humpston, and Henry J. Jackson - Models of Schizophrenia. A Selective Review of Genetic, Neuropharmacological, Cognitive, and Social Approaches / Megan Ichinose and Sohee Park - Understanding the Impact of Mental Health Stigma and the Role of Clinicians as Allies / Katherine Nieweglowski, Sang Qin, Deysi Paniagua, Patrick W. Corrigan - Culture and psychosis in clinical practice / G. E. Jarvis, Srividya Iyer, Lisa Andermann and Kenneth Fung - The recovery model and psychosis / Bethany Leonhardt, Jay Hamm and Paul Lysaker - Section Two: Assessment. Assessment in psychosis / Rebecca Kelly, Christopher Shoulder and Vaughan Bell - Negative symptoms and their assessment in schizophrenia and related disorders / Jack Blanchard, LeeAnn Shan, Alexandra Andrea, Christina Savage, Ann M. Kring and Lauren Weittenhiller - Assessing social and non-social cognition in schizophrenia and related disorders / Amy Pinkham and Johanna Badcock - Assessing social functioning across the life course of psychosis / Helen Stain and Jone Bjornestad - Trauma, psychosis and post-traumatic stress disorder / Amy Hardy, Irene van de Giessen and David P. G. van den Berg - Effectively Assessing Sleep and Circadian Rhythms in Psychosis / Jan Cosgrave, Elizabeth Klingaman and Philip Gehrman - Benefits, assessment and preferences of physical activity in psychosis / Shuichi Suetani and Joseph Firth -

Screening and assessment of substance use disorder in psychosis / Kim T. Mueser - Section Three: Linking Assessment to Treatment. Clinical case formulation / Katherine Berry, Gillian Haddock and Georgie Paulik - Section Four: Therapies. Cognitive Behavioural Therapies for Psychosis / Louise Johns, Louise Isham, and Rachel Manser - Third Wave CBT Interventions for Psychosis / Lyn Ellett and Jessica Kingston - Cognitive remediation to improve functional outcome / Alice Medalia and Alice Saperstein - Promoting psychosocial functioning and recovery in schizophrenia spectrum and other psychotic disorders / Olga Santesteban-Echarri, Simon Rice, Cesar Gonzalez Blanch and Mario Alvarez-Jimenez - Trauma therapies in psychosis / David P. G. van den Berg, Irene van de Giessen and Amy Hardy - Better sleep: Evidence-based interventions / Felicity Waite and Bryony Sheaves - Get moving: physical activity and exercise for mental health / Hamish Fibbins, Oscar Lederman, Simon Rosenbaum - Treating comorbid substance use and psychosis / Amanda L. Baker, Alexandra M.J. Denham, Sonja Pohlman, and Kristen McCarter - A brief guide to medications for psychosis / Anthony Harris - Getting in early: Early intervention services for psychosis / Jesse Gates and Eóin Killackey - Section Five: New Directions in Research and Practice. Beyond belief: new approaches to the treatment of paranoia / Philippa Anne Garety, Thomas Ward, and Mar Rus-Calafell - Being a scientist-practitioner in the field of psychosis: Experiences from voices clinics / Georgie Paulik, Neil Thomas, Evie Glasshouse, and Mark Hayward - The therapeutic use of digital technologies in psychosis / Imogen Bell, Michelle Lim and Neil Thomas - Tracking language in real time in psychosis / Terje B. Holmlund, Taylor L. Fedechko, Brita Elvevåg and Alex S. Cohen - Integrating lived

	experience perspectives into clinical practice / Catherine van Zelst.
LC Subjects	Psychoses.
Other Subjects	Psychotic Disorders
	Psychoses.
Notes	Includes bibliographical references and index.
Additional formats	ebook version: 9780128150139

Assessment of feigned cognitive impairment: a neuropsychological perspective

LCCN	2021014065
Type of material	Book
Main title	Assessment of feigned cognitive impairment: a neuropsychological perspective / edited by Kyle Brauer Boone.
Edition	Second edition.
Published/Produced	New York: The Guilford Press, [2021]
ISBN	9781462545551 (hardcover)
LC classification	RC386.6.N48 A86 2021
Related names	Boone, K. B. (Kyle Brauer) editor.
Summary	"The go-to resource for clinical and forensic practice has now been significantly revised with 85% new material, reflecting the tremendous growth of the field. Leading authorities synthesize the state of the science on symptom feigning in cognitive testing and present evidence-based recommendations for distinguishing between credible and noncredible performance. A wide range of performance validity tests (PVTs) and symptom validity tests (SVTs) are critically reviewed and guidelines provided for applying them across differing cognitive domains and medical, neurological, and psychiatric conditions. The book also covers validity testing in forensic settings and with special populations"-- Provided by publisher.
	"The go-to resource for clinical and forensic practice has now been significantly revised with 85% new material, reflecting the tremendous growth of the field. Leading authorities synthesize the state of the

science on symptom feigning in cognitive testing and present evidence-based recommendations for distinguishing between credible and noncredible performance. A wide range of performance validity tests (PVTs) and symptom validity tests (SVTs) are critically reviewed and guidelines provided for applying them across differing cognitive domains and medical, neurological, and psychiatric conditions. The book also covers validity testing in forensic settings and with particular populations, such as ethnic and linguistic minority group members. New to This Edition *Numerous new authors, a greatly expanded range of topics, and the latest data throughout. *"Clinical primer" chapter on how to select and interpret appropriate PVTs. *Chapters on methods for validity testing in visual spatial, processing speed, and language domains and with cognitive screening instruments and personality inventories. *Chapter on methods for interpreting multiple PVTs in combination. *Chapters on additional populations (military personnel, children and adolescents) and clinical problems (dementia, somatoform/conversion disorder). *Chapters on research methods for validating PVTs, base rates of feigned mild traumatic brain injury, and more. "-- Provided by publisher.

Contents I. Performance and Symptom Validity Tests - 1. Clinician's Guide to Navigating Performance Validity Testing, Maria E. Cottingham - 2. Design Methods in Neuropsychological Performance Validity, Symptom Validity, and Malingering Research, Ryan W. Schroeder, Kyle Brauer Boone, & Glenn J. Larrabee - 3. Forced-Choice Performance Validity Tests, Ryan W. Schroeder & Phillip K. Martin - 4. Alternatives to Forced-Choice Performance Validity Tests, Stephen R. Nitch, Alexis S. Rosen, Laurel A. Mattos, Scott Roye, & David M. Glassmire - 5. Intelligence Tests as Performance Validity Measures, Natalie Sobel, Talin Babikian, &

Kyle Brauer Boone - 6. Performance Validity Tests in Cognitive Screening Instruments and Computerized Assessment Tools, Patrick Armistead-Jehle & Robert D. Shura - 7. Embedded Performance Validity Scores in Standard Memory Tests, Bradley N. Axelrod, Justin B. Miller, & Jennifer LaBuda - 8. Validity Indicators within Executive Function Measures: Use and Limits in Detection of Response Validity, Nathaniel W. Nelson, Catherine Lee, & Jerry J. Sweet - 9. Motor and Sensory Tests as Measures of Performance Validity, Ginger Arnold & Kyle Brauer Boone - 10. The Use of Visual Spatial Performance Validity Tests in Detecting Noncredible Performance, Douglas M. Whiteside, Lauren E. Piper, Michael R. Basso, & Kyle Brauer Boone - 11. Information Processing Speed Tests as Performance Validity Tests, Laszlo A. Erdodi & Jonathan D. Lichtenstein - 12. Language Tests as Performance Validity Tests, Phillip K. Martin & Ryan W. Schroeder - 13. Effects of Premorbid Ability, Neuropsychological Impairment, and Invalid Test Performance on the Frequency of Low Scores, Martin L. Rohling, Jennifer Langhinrichsen-Rohling, & John E. Meyers - 14. Interpretation of Data from Multiple Performance Validity Tests, Jeremy J. Davis - 15. Using the MMPI-2-RF as an Aid in the Detection of Noncredible Neurocognitive Presentations, Maria E. Cottingham, Kyle Brauer Boone, Hope E. Goldberg, Tara L. Victor, Michelle A. Zeller, Medina R. Baumgart, J. Brandon Birath, & Matthew J. Wright - 16. Utility of the Personality Assessment Inventory in Evaluating Symptom Validity in the Context of Neuropsychological Evaluation, Owen J. Gaasedelen, Douglas M. Whiteside, & Kyle Brauer Boone - II. Use of Performance Validity Tests in Various Populations - 17. Base Rates of Feigned Mild Traumatic Brain Injury, Kyle Brauer Boone, Pavel Litvin, & Tara L. Victor - 18. Noncredible Presentations in Neuropsychological Assessment of

Bibliography

Pain- and Fatigue-Related Disorders: Clinical and Research Implications, Julie A. Suhr & Andrew Bryant - 19. The Impact of Psychotic, Depressive, Bipolar, Obsessive-Compulsive, and Anxiety Disorders on Performance Validity Test Results, Hope E. Goldberg & J. Brandon Birath - 20. Performance Validity in Somatoform/Conversion Disorders, Factitious Disorder, and Malingering: Do We Need a New Diagnostic Schema?, Kyle Brauer Boone - 21. Identification of Feigned Intellectual Disability, Tara L. Victor & Kyle Brauer Boone - 22. Performance Validity Testing in Patients with Dementia, Kirsty E. Bortnik & Andy C. Dean - 23. Performance Validity Tests in the Epilepsy Clinic, Daniel L. Drane, David J. Williamson, Kelsey Hewitt, & Taylor Jordan - 24. Use of Performance Validity Tests and Symptom Validity Tests in Assessment of Specific Learning Disorders and Attention-Deficit/Hyperactivity Disorder, Allyson G. Harrison, Grace Jin Lee, & Julie A. Suhr - 25. Toxic Mold Syndrome and Multiple Chemical Sensitivity: The Continued Search for a Causal Link to Neuropsychological Functioning, Robert J. McCaffrey & Julie K. Lynch - 26. The Use of Performance Validity Tests in Ethnic-Minority and Non-English-Dominant Populations, Xavier F. Salazar, Po H. Lu, & Kyle Brauer Boone - 27. Performance/Symptom Validity Test Use with Active Duty Service Members and Veterans, Patrick Armistead-Jehle, Douglas B. Cooper, Heather G. Belanger, Jason R. Soble, & Nathanial W. Nelson - 28. Validity Assessment in Pediatric Populations, Alison M. Colbert, Emily C. Maxwell, & Michael W. Kirkwood - 29. Assessment of Feigned Cognitive Impairment in Criminal Forensic Neuropsychological Settings, Robert L. Denney & Rachel L. Fazio - Index.

LC Subjects

Neuropsychological tests.
Cognition--Testing.

Other Subjects	Cognition disorders--Diagnosis. Factitious disorders--Diagnosis. Malingering--Diagnosis. Psychology / Neuropsychology Psychology / Forensic Psychology
Notes	Includes bibliographical references and index.

Behavioral science

LCCN	2019043679
Type of material	Book
Personal name	Fadem, Barbara, author.
Main title	Behavioral science / Barbara Fadem.
Edition	Eighth edition.
Published/Produced	Philadelphia: Wolters Kluwer, [2021]
ISBN	9781975118365 softbound
LC classification	RC457.2
Summary	"Offering current coverage of behavioral science, psychiatry, epidemiology, and related topics, BRS Behavioral Science, Eighth Edition, prepares students to rapidly recall key information on the mind-body relationship and confidently apply that knowledge on exams and in practice. The popular BRS format presents essential information in a succinct, streamlined approach preferred by today's busy students, accompanied by hundreds of USMLE-style review questions with detailed answers and explanations to help strengthen students' exam readiness"-- Provided by publisher.
Contents	The beginning of life: pregnancy through preschool - School age, adolescence, special issues of development, and adulthood - Aging, death, and bereavement - Genetics, anatomy, and biochemistry of behavior - Biological assessment of patients with psychiatric symptoms - Psychoanalytic theory and defense mechanisms - Learning theory --Clinical assessment of patients with behavioral symptoms - Substance-related disorders - Typical sleep and sleep-wake disorders - Schizophrenia spectrum and other psychotic disorders - Depressive disorders and

	bipolar and related disorders - Anxiety disorders, obsessive-compulsive and related disorders, somatic symptom disorders, and trauma and stressor-related disorders - Psychiatric disorders in children - Biologic therapies: psychopharmacology - Psychological therapies The family, culture, and illness - Sexuality - Aggression and abuse - The physician-patient relationship - Psychosomatic medicine - Legal and ethical issues in medicine - Health care in the United States - Medical epidemiology - Statistical analyses.
Other Subjects	Behavioral Sciences Behavior

Clinical consult to psychiatric mental health management for nurse practitioners

LCCN	2020037434
Type of material	Book
Personal name	Rhoads, Jacqueline, 1948- author.
Uniform title	Clinical consult to psychiatric nursing for advanced practice
Main title	Clinical consult to psychiatric mental health management for nurse practitioners / Jacqueline Rhoads.
Edition	Second edition.
Published/Produced	New York, NY: Springer Publishing Company, LLC, [2021]
Description	1 online resource
ISBN	9780826161840 (ebook) (paperback)
LC classification	RC440
Summary	"Provides "what to do next" guidelines when working with and beginning the treatment of a patient with a mental health disorder. Compiled by expert practitioners in psychiatric care, this work provides an overview of the management of the major Diagnostic and Statistical Manual of Mental Disorders, Fifth Edition (American Psychiatric Association, 2013) disorders across the life span and

Contents	delivers complete clinical guidelines for their diagnosis, treatment options, and psychopharmacologic management"-- Provided by publisher. The psychiatric interview and diagnosis - Psychotherapeutic management - Behavioral therapy, cognitive-behavioral therapy, and psychoanalysis - The relationship of psychopharmacology to neurotransmitters, receptors, signal transduction, and second messengers - Clinical neuroanatomy of the brain - Principles of pharmacokinetics and pharmacodynamics - Principles and management of psychiatric emergencies - Behavioral and psychological disorders in the elderly - Substance use disorders - Psychotic disorders - Mood disorders - Anxiety disorders - Obsessive-compulsive disorders - Dissociative disorders - Sexual dysfunction - Feeding and eating disorders - Sleep disorders - Personality disorders - Neurodevelopmental disorders - Drug monographs.
Other Subjects	Mental Disorders--nursing Mental Disorders--therapy Psychiatric Nursing--methods Nurse Practitioners--standards Psychopharmacology--methods
Notes	Preceded by Clinical consult to psychiatric nursing for advanced practice / Jacqueline Rhoads, Patrick J.M. Murphy. [2015]. Includes bibliographical references and index.
Additional formats	Print version: Rhoads, Jacqueline, 1948- Clinical consult to psychiatric mental health management for nurse practitioners Second edition. New York, NY: Springer Publishing Company, LLC, [2021] 9780826161833 (DLC) 2020037433

Clinical consult to psychiatric mental health management for nurse practitioners

LCCN	2020037433
Type of material	Book
Personal name	Rhoads, Jacqueline, 1948- author.

Uniform title	Clinical consult to psychiatric nursing for advanced practice
Main title	Clinical consult to psychiatric mental health management for nurse practitioners / Jacqueline Rhoads, PhD, ACNP-BC, ANP-C, PMHNP-BE, CNL C, FAANP.
Edition	Second edition.
Published/Produced	New York, NY: Springer Publishing Company, LLC, [2021]
Description	xix, 609 pages; 26 cm
ISBN	9780826161833 (paperback) (ebook)
LC classification	RC440 .R485 2021
Summary	"Provides "what to do next" guidelines when working with and beginning the treatment of a patient with a mental health disorder. Compiled by expert practitioners in psychiatric care, this work provides an overview of the management of the major Diagnostic and Statistical Manual of Mental Disorders, Fifth Edition (American Psychiatric Association, 2013) disorders across the life span and delivers complete clinical guidelines for their diagnosis, treatment options, and psycho-pharmacologic management"-- Provided by publisher.
Contents	The psychiatric interview and diagnosis - Psychotherapeutic management - Behavioral therapy, cognitive-behavioral therapy, and psychoanalysis - The relationship of psychopharmacology to neurotransmitters, receptors, signal transduction, and second messengers - Clinical neuroanatomy of the brain - Principles of pharmacokinetics and pharmacodynamics - Principles and management of psychiatric emergencies - Behavioral and psychological disorders in the elderly - Substance use disorders - Psychotic disorders - Mood disorders - Anxiety disorders - Obsessive-compulsive disorders - Dissociative disorders - Sexual dysfunction - Feeding and eating disorders - Sleep disorders -

Other Subjects	Personality disorders - Neurodevelopmental disorders - Drug monographs. Mental Disorders--nursing Mental Disorders--therapy Psychiatric Nursing--methods Nurse Practitioners--standards Psychopharmacology--methods
Notes	Preceded by Clinical consult to psychiatric nursing for advanced practice / Jacqueline Rhoads, Patrick J.M. Murphy. [2015]. Includes bibliographical references and index.
Additional formats	Online version: Rhoads, Jacqueline, 1948- Clinical consult to psychiatric mental health management for nurse practitioners Second edition. New York, NY: Springer Publishing Company, LLC, [2021] 9780826161840 (DLC) 2020037434

Clinical handbook of psychological disorders: a step-by-step treatment manual

LCCN	2021014995
Type of material	Book
Main title	Clinical handbook of psychological disorders: a step-by-step treatment manual / edited by David H. Barlow.
Edition	Sixth edition.
Published/Produced	New York: The Guilford Press, [2021]
ISBN	9781462547043 (hardcover)
LC classification	RC489.B4 C584 2021
Related names	Barlow, David H., editor.
Summary	"Now in a revised and expanded sixth edition, this is the leading text on evidence-based treatments for frequently encountered mental health problems. David H. Barlow has assembled preeminent experts to present their respective approaches in step-by-step detail, including extended case examples. Each chapter provides state-of-the-art information on the disorder at hand, explains the conceptual and empirical bases of intervention, and addresses the most pressing question asked by students and

practitioners--"How do I do it?" Concise chapter introductions from Barlow highlight the unique features of each treatment and enhance the book's utility for teaching and training. New to This Edition *Existing chapters thoroughly revised to incorporate the latest empirical findings and clinical practices. *Chapter on "process-based therapy," a new third-wave approach for social anxiety. *Chapter on transdiagnostic treatment of self-injurious thoughts and behaviors. *Chapter on chronic pain"-- Provided by publisher.

Contents

Machine generated contents note: 1. Panic Disorder and Agoraphobia, Michelle G. Craske, Kate Wolitzky-Taylor, & David H. Barlow - 2. Posttraumatic Stress Disorder, Candice M. Monson, Philippe Shnaider, & Kathleen M. Chard - 3. Social Anxiety: A Process-Based Treatment Approach, Idan M. Aderka & Stefan G. Hofmann - 4. Obsessive-Compulsive Disorder, Martin E. Franklin & Edna B. Foa - 5. Generalized Anxiety Disorder: An Acceptance-Based Behavioral Therapy, Lizabeth Roemer, Elizabeth H. Eustis, & Susan M. Orsillo - 6. Emotional Disorders: A Unified Protocol for Transdiagnostic Treatment, Laura A. Payne, Kristen K. Ellard, Todd J. Farchione, & David H. Barlow - 7. Cognitive Therapy for Depression, Jeffrey E. Young, Erin F. Ward-Ciesielski, Jayne L. Rygh, Arthur D. Weinberger, & Aaron T. Beck - 8. Interpersonal Psychotherapy for Depression, Kathryn L. Bleiberg & John C. Markowitz - 9. Behavioral Activation for Depression, Sona Dimidjian, Christopher R. Martell, Ruth Herman-Dunn, & Samuel Hubley - 10. Borderline Personality Disorder, Andrada D. Neacsiu, Noga Zerubavel, K. Maria Nylocks, & Marsha M. Linehan - 11. Addressing Self-Injurious Thoughts and Behaviors within the Context of Transdiagnostic Treatment for Emotional Disorders, Kate H. Bentley, Joseph S. Maimone, & Matthew K. Nock - 12. Bipolar Disorder, David J. Miklowitz - 13.

	Schizophrenia and Other Psychotic Disorders, Nicholas Tarrier & Katherine Berry - 14. Alcohol Use Disorders, Barbara S. McCrady & Elizabeth E. Epstein - 15. Substance Use Disorders, Stephen T. Higgins, Sarah H. Heil, & Kelly R. Peck - 16. Sleep Disturbance, Katherine A. Kaplan & Allison G. Harvey - 17. Cognitive-Behavioral Therapy for Chronic Pain, John D. Otis - 18. Eating Disorders: A Transdiagnostic Protocol, Zafra Cooper & Rebecca Murphy - 19. Couple Distress, Andrew Christensen, Jennifer G. Wheeler, Brian D. Doss, & Neil S. Jacobson - Author Index - Subject Index.
LC Subjects	Behavior therapy--Handbooks, manuals, etc.
	Medical protocols--Handbooks, manuals, etc.
Other Subjects	Psychology / Psychopathology / General
	Psychology / Clinical Psychology
Notes	Includes bibliographical references and index.

Clinical manual of youth addictive disorders

LCCN	2019033776
Type of material	Book
Main title	Clinical manual of youth addictive disorders / edited by Yifrah Kaminer, Ken C. Winters.
Published/Produced	Washington, DC: American Psychiatric Association Publishing, [2020]
Description	1 online resource
ISBN	9781615372812 (ebook)
	(paperback)
LC classification	RJ506.D78
Related titles	Preceded by (work): Clinical manual of adolescent substance abuse treatment.
Related names	Kaminer, Yifrah, 1951- editor.
	Winters, Ken C., editor.
	American Psychiatric Association Publishing, issuing body.
Summary	"This long-awaited follow-up to the classic text Clinical Manual of Adolescent Substance Abuse Treatment presents the latest research on substance use and substance use disorders (SUDs) in

adolescents 12-18 and emerging adults 18-25 years of age. This new manual offers a substantive update of the previous manual's 16 chapters, offering 7 additional chapters devoted to important new topics, such as pediatric primary care assessment and intervention, electronic tools, specific substances (e.g., cannabis, opioids, alcohol), and much more. Psychiatrists, psychologists, social workers, and substance abuse specialists, as well as applied researchers and public health professionals, will find this new manual a research-rich and clinically compelling resource for understanding disease course, prevention, diagnosis, substance-specific interventions, co-occurring disorders, and issues related to special populations"-- Provided by publisher.

Contents Diagnosis, Epidemiology, and Course of Youth Substance Use and Use Disorders / Gerald Montano, D.O., Tammy Chung, Ph.D. - Prevention of Substance Use and Substance Use Disorders / Lawrence M. Scheier, Ph.D., Richard Catalano, Ph.D., Ken C. Winters, Ph.D. - Screening and Assessing Youth With Substance Use Disorder / Ken C. Winters, Ph.D., Randy Stinchfield, Ph.D., Andria M. Botzet, M.A. - Primary Care and Pediatric Settings: SCREENING, BRIEF INTERVENTION, AND REFERRAL TO TREATMENT (SBIRT) / Areej Hassan, M.D., M.P.H., Sion K. Harris, Ph.D., John Rogers Knight, M.D. - Bioassays and Detection of Substances of Abuse in Youth / Albert J. Arias, M.D., Wendy Welch, M.D., C.P.E., Yifrah Kaminer, M.D., M.B.A. - Placement Criteria and Integrated Treatment Services for Youth With Substance Use Disorders / Marc Fishman, M.D. - Youth Alcohol Use / Robert Miranda, Jr., Ph.D., Ryan W. Carpenter, Ph.D. - Pharmacological Treatment of Youth Tobacco Use / Grace Kong, Ph.D. - Youth Cannabis Use / Christian Thurstone, M.D., Yifrah Kaminer, M.D., M.B.A. - Youth Opioid Use / Christopher J.

Hammond, M.D., Ph.D., Brian Hendrickson, M.D., Marc Fishman, M.D. - Youth Club, Prescription, and Over-the-Counter Drug Use / Charles Albert Whitmore, M.D., M.P.H., Christian Hopfer, M.D. - Continuity of Care for Abstinence and Harm Reduction / Yifrah Kaminer, M.D., M.B.A., Mark D. Godley, Ph.D., Ken C. Winters, Ph.D., Kara Bagot, M.D. - Brief Motivational Interventions, Cognitive-Behavioral Therapy, and Contingency Management / Anthony Spirito, Ph.D., A.B.P.P., Yifrah Kaminer, M.D., M.B.A., Kimberly H. McManama O'Brien, Ph.D., L.I.C.S.W. - Family and Community-Based Therapies / Molly Bobek, L.C.S.W., Susan H. Godley, Rh.D., Aaron Hogue, Ph.D. - Twelve-Step and Mutual-Help Programs / John F. Kelly, Ph.D., Alexandra W. Abry, B.A., Nilofar Fallah-Sohy, B.S. - Electronic Tools and Resources for Assessing and Treating Youth Substance Use Disorders / Rachel Gonzales-Castaneda, Ph.D., M.P.H., Kyle C. McCarthy, M.S., Briana Thrasher, B.A. - Assessment and Treatment of Co-occurring Internalizing Disorders: DEPRESSION, ANXIETY DISORDERS, AND PTSD / Yifrah Kaminer, M.D., M.B.A., Kristyn Zajac, Ph.D., Ken C. Winters, Ph.D. - Assessment and Treatment of Co-occurring Suicidal Behavior / David B. Goldston, Ph.D., Angela M. Tunno, Ph.D., John F. Curry, Ph.D., Karen C. Wells, Ph.D., Michelle Roley-Roberts, Ph.D. - Assessment and Treatment of Comorbid Psychotic Disorders: BIPOLAR DISORDER, SCHIZOPHRENIA, AND DRUG-INDUCED PSYCHOTIC DISORDERS / Kara S. Bagot, M.D., Robert Milin, M.D., F.R.C.P.C., Desiree Shapiro, M.D., Daphna Finn, M.D., Shavon Moore, M.D. - Assessment and Treatment of Co-occurring Externalizing Disorders: ATTENTION-DEFICIT/HYPERACTIVITY DISORDER AND DISRUPTIVE BEHAVIOR DISORDERS / Martha J. Ignaszewski, M.D., K.A.H. Mirza, M.B., F.R.C.P.C., Oscar G. Bukstein, M.D.,

	M.P.H. - Behavioral Addictions: GAMBLING DISORDER AND INTERNET GAMING DISORDER / Luis C. Farhat, M.D., Jeffrey Derevensky, Ph.D., Marc N. Potenza, M.D., Ph.D. - Management of Youth With Substance Use Disorders in the Juvenile Justice System / Kristyn Zajac, Ph.D., Tess K. Drazdowski, Ph.D., Ashli J. Sheidow, Ph.D. - Maternal Substance Use in Pregnancy / Amy M. Johnson, M.D., F.A.C.O.G., Courtney Townsel, M.D., M.Sc., F.A.C.O.G
Other Subjects	Substance-Related Disorders--diagnosis
	Substance-Related Disorders--therapy
	Behavior, Addictive
	Comorbidity
	Adolescent
Notes	Includes bibliographical references and index.
Additional formats	Print version: Clinical manual of youth addictive disorders Washington, DC: American Psychiatric Association Publishing, [2020] 9781615372362 (DLC) 2019033775

Clinical psychology in the mental health inpatient setting: international perspectives

LCCN	2019010598
Type of material	Book
Main title	Clinical psychology in the mental health inpatient setting: international perspectives / [edited by] Meidan Turel, Michael Siglag, and Alexander Grinshpoon.
Published/Produced	New York: Routledge, 2020.
Description	1 online resource
ISBN	9780429464584 (E-book)
LC classification	RC480.5
Related names	Turel, Meidan, editor.
	Siglag, Michael, editor.
	Grinshpoon, Alexander, editor.
Contents	Therapy beyond walls: the clinical psychologist's multi-level work in the psychiatric ward / Mark Andrew McFetridge - The clinical psychologist in an

open inpatient setting: a psychoanalytic perspective / Marilyn Charles - Clinical psychologists in Australian in-patient mental health units: enhancing effectiveness and relevance with a human rights focus / Peter Walker and Sophie Li - Ethical challenges for psychologists providing inpatient mental health care / Heidi Camerlengo - The benefit of behavior support plans in psychiatric inpatient settings / Jimmy I. Kim and Peter J. D'Amacio - Three dynamic roles of the clinical psychologist on the acute closed psychiatric ward / Amit Fachler - The development of a recovery-oriented tool for work with patients in the closed forensic ward / Enav Or-Gordon - On trying to stay sane in insane places: a personal account of a clinical psychologist's challenges on the psychiatric inpatient ward / Jim Geekie - A path taken: a psychologist's professional journey within the psychiatric inpatient system / Michael Siglag - All brief therapy is not created equal: the contribution of psychology to short-stay mental health inpatient admissions / Manish Parswani and Malcolm W. Stewart - Continuity model of care: working across acute inpatient to community-based clinical psychology / Kim Griffiths, Hannah Green, and Suzie Lemmey - Cognitive behavioral therapy for psychosis on the inpatient unit: the role of the clinical psychologist / Sally E. Riggs - Psychotherapy in an in-patient ward: a clinical psychologist's use of psychoanalytic informed work with adult survivors of childhood trauma / Beatriz S. Curtis - Mentalization and psychotherapy: a way to understand patient violence on the psychiatric inpatient unit / Dione Johnson-Williams - The clinical psychologist's work in a forensic psychiatry ward: building a transitional space for individuals with mental disorders who committed crimes / Hilik Peri - Psychodynamic psychological testing in the mental health inpatient setting: a way of listening, learning, and holding patients and psychotherapists / Christina

	Biedermann, Jeremy Ridenour, and Spencer E. Biel - "Listening to the music of the mind": the uses of psychological assessment in the diagnosis of psychotic disorders in a state psychiatric center / Paul Saks - The role of psychological testing in an inpatient psychiatric setting: a mentalizing approach / Shweta Sharma & Patricia Daza - A clinical psychology intern's experience of training in an inpatient unit: no training wheels / Daria Mamon - The benefits and challenges of clinical psychology internships in psychiatric inpatient settings / Valerie Sims - The most difficult lesson: the impact of patient suicide on training in an inpatient psychiatric hospital / Patricia Daza and Shweta Sharma - An intern's experience on an acute closed ward: "from a shadow to a bird": the psychotherapeutic process of Berry / Karin Reddie - Weaving with a relational thread: the clinical psychologist's use of empathy in work in the mental health inpatient setting / Meidan Turel - Concluding thoughts: past and present trends, future directions / Michael Siglag.
Other Subjects	Psychotherapy--methods
	Mental Disorders--therapy
	Psychiatric Department, Hospital
	Inpatients--psychology
Notes	Includes bibliographical references and index.
Additional formats	Print version: Clinical psychology in the mental health inpatient setting New York, NY: Routledge, 2019 9781138612716 (DLC) 2019008482

Co-occurring mental illness and substance use disorders: evidence-based integrative treatment and multicultural application

LCCN	2021047453
Type of material	Book
Main title	Co-occurring mental illness and substance use disorders: evidence-based integrative treatment and multicultural application / edited by Tricia L. Chandler, Fredrick Dombrowski, Tara G. Matthews.
Published/Produced	New York, NY: Routledge, 2022.

Description	1 online resource
ISBN	9781000562101 (epub)
	9781003220916 (ebook)
	(hardback)
	(paperback)
LC classification	RC480
Related names	Chandler, Tricia L., editor.
	Dombrowski, Fredrick, editor.
	Matthews, Tara G., editor.
Summary	"This textbook details how mental health and addiction are interconnected through childhood trauma, how this affects neurobiology and neuropsychology, and the need for an integrated whole-person treatment for those of diverse backgrounds to enhance treatment outcomes. Using an integrative pedagogy, the book helps readers broaden their understanding of co-occurring disorders through case studies, learning objectives, key terms, quiz questions, suggested resources, and references. By linking to previous knowledge and suggesting practical applications, each chapter provides clear direction for learning more about each treatment approach, diagnosis, and population discussed within the multi-cultural and biopsychosocial perspective. Co-occurring Mental Illness and Substance Use Disorders will help graduate students in both substance use and mental health counseling make sense of integrative treatment with co-occurring disorders"-- Provided by publisher.
Contents	Trauma, PTSD, substance use, & neuroscience - Mood & anxiety disorders - Psychotic disorders and co-occurring substance use disorders - Co-occurring personality and substance use disorders - Attention deficit hyperactive disorder - Process use disorders - Women with co-occurring disorders - Men with co-occurring disorders - Adolescence with co-occurring disorders - Co-occurring disorders among the older adult population - LGBTQIA and co-occurring disorders - Multicultural perspectives in co-occurring

	treatment - Assessment of co-occurring disorders, levels of care and ASAM requirements - Recovery programming: 12-steps, cognitive behavioral therapy and motivational interviewing - Biological approaches: pharmacotherapy, MAT, orthomolecular psychiatry, & nutrition - Consciousness: spirituality, mindfulness, meditation and mindfulness-based therapies - Creative arts & somatic therapies: psychodrama, eye movement desensitization regulation & body/mind therapies - How East met West: the emergence of energy psychology as a body/mind approach - Animal assisted therapies.
LC Subjects	Mental illness--Treatment--Textbooks. Substance abuse--Treatment--Textbooks. Psychotherapy--Textbooks.
Notes	Includes bibliographical references and index.
Additional formats	Print version: Co-occurring mental illness and substance use disorders New York, NY: Routledge, 2022 9781032116525 (DLC) 2021047452

Co-occurring mental illness and substance use disorders: evidence-based integrative treatment and multicultural application

LCCN	2021047452
Type of material	Book
Main title	Co-occurring mental illness and substance use disorders: evidence-based integrative treatment and multicultural application / edited by Tricia L. Chandler, Fredrick Dombrowski, Tara G. Matthews.
Published/Produced	New York, NY: Routledge, Taylor & Francis Group, 2022.
Description	xiv, 270 pages: illustrations; 26 cm
ISBN	9781032116518 (paperback) 9781032116525 (hardback) (ebook)
LC classification	RC480 .C565 2022
Related names	Chandler, Tricia L., editor. Dombrowski, Fredrick, editor. Matthews, Tara G., editor.

Summary	"This textbook details how mental health and addiction are interconnected through childhood trauma, how this affects neurobiology and neuropsychology, and the need for an integrated whole-person treatment for those of diverse backgrounds to enhance treatment outcomes. Using an integrative pedagogy, the book helps readers broaden their understanding of co-occurring disorders through case studies, learning objectives, key terms, quiz questions, suggested resources, and references. By linking to previous knowledge and suggesting practical applications, each chapter provides clear direction for learning more about each treatment approach, diagnosis, and population discussed within the multi-cultural and biopsychosocial perspective. Co-occurring Mental Illness and Substance Use Disorders will help graduate students in both substance use and mental health counseling make sense of integrative treatment with co-occurring disorders"-- Provided by publisher.
Contents	Trauma, PTSD, substance use, & neuroscience - Mood & anxiety disorders - Psychotic disorders and co-occurring substance use disorders - Co-occurring personality and substance use disorders - Attention deficit hyperactive disorder - Process use disorders - Women with co-occurring disorders - Men with co-occurring disorders - Adolescence with co-occurring disorders - Co-occurring disorders among the older adult population - LGBTQIA and co-occurring disorders - Multicultural perspectives in co-occurring treatment - Assessment of co-occurring disorders, levels of care and ASAM requirements - Recovery programming: 12-steps, cognitive behavioral therapy and motivational interviewing - Biological approaches: pharmacotherapy, MAT, orthomolecular psychiatry, & nutrition - Consciousness: spirituality, mindfulness, meditation and mindfulness-based therapies - Creative arts & somatic therapies: psychodrama, eye movement desensitization

	regulation & body/mind therapies - How East met West: the emergence of energy psychology as a body/mind approach - Animal assisted therapies.
LC Subjects	Mental illness--Treatment--Textbooks.
	Substance abuse--Treatment--Textbooks.
	Psychotherapy--Textbooks.
Notes	Includes bibliographical references and index.
Additional formats	Online version: Co-occurring mental illness and substance use disorders New York, NY: Routledge, 2022 9781003220916 (DLC) 2021047453

Dealing with psychotic disorders

LCCN	2019034014
Type of material	Book
Personal name	Miller, Marie-Therese, author.
Main title	Dealing with psychotic disorders / By Marie-Therese Miller, Ph. D.
Published/Produced	San Diego, CA: ReferencePoint Press, [2020]
ISBN	9781682827932 (hardcover)
	(eBook)
LC classification	RC512 .M55 2020
Summary	"Those with psychotic disorders can see or hear things that do not exist in reality. Dealing with Psychotic Disorders explores what these disorders are like, how they affect people's lives, and today's best treatment options"-- Provided by publisher.
LC Subjects	Psychoses.
	Psychoses--Treatment.
	Psychoses in adolescence.
Notes	Includes bibliographical references and index.
Intended Audience	Grades 10-12 (ReferencePoint Press.)
Additional formats	Online version: Miller, Ph. D., Marie-Therese, 1960- Dealing with psychotic disorders San Diego: ReferencePoint Press, 2020. 9781682827949 (DLC) 2019034015
Series	Dealing with mental disorders

Dealing with psychotic disorders

LCCN	2019034015
Type of material	Book
Personal name	Miller, Marie-Therese, author.
Main title	Dealing with psychotic disorders / By Marie-Therese Miller, Ph. D.
Published/Produced	San Diego, CA: ReferencePoint Press, [2020]
Description	1 online resource.
ISBN	9781682827949 (pdf)
	(hardcover)
LC classification	RC512
Summary	"Those with psychotic disorders can see or hear things that do not exist in reality. Dealing with Psychotic Disorders explores what these disorders are like, how they affect people's lives, and today's best treatment options"-- Provided by publisher.
LC Subjects	Psychoses.
	Psychoses--Treatment.
	Psychoses in adolescence.
Notes	Includes bibliographical references and index.
Intended Audience	Grades 10-12 (ReferencePoint Press.)
Additional formats	Print version: Miller, Marie-Therese. Dealing with psychotic disorders San Diego, CA: ReferencePoint Press, [2020] 9781682827932 (DLC) 2019034014
Series	Dealing with mental disorders

Decriminalizing mental illness

LCCN	2020031748
Type of material	Book
Main title	Decriminalizing mental illness / edited by Katherine Warburton, Stephen M. Stahl.
Published/Produced	Cambridge; New York, NY: Cambridge University Press, 2021.
ISBN	9781108826952 (paperback)
	(ebook)
LC classification	RA1148
Related names	Warburton, Katherine D., editor.
	Stahl, Stephen M., 1951- editor.

Summary	"The history of serious mental illness (SMI) is grim, from a cultural as well as a treatment perspective. The conditions of individuals with psychotic disorders have swung, like a pendulum, from institutional neglect to community neglect and back again over the past several hundred years. At the core of treatment failure is a failure in mental health policy and funding, with the result usually framed as the degree of human institutionalization in jails, prisons and asylums. In the middle of the 19th century, institutions designed to deliver moral treatment were considered the humane answer to care properly for the SMI population. By the mid- 20th century, those same, now overcrowded, institutions were blamed for the horrible conditions of mistreatment of individuals with SMI. Now, as we approach the middle of the 21st century, deinstitutionalization (the answer to the cruel asylums) is purportedly at fault for homelessness, lack of treatment, and criminalization. As the pendulum swings, we are hearing cries to "bring back" the asylums"-- Provided by publisher.
Other Subjects	Forensic Psychiatry--methods
	Commitment of Mentally Ill--legislation & jurisprudence
	Criminal Law--methods
	Institutionalization
	Psychotic Disorders--therapy
	Insanity Defense
Notes	Includes bibliographical references and index.
Additional formats	Online version: Decriminalizing mental illness. Cambridge; New York, NY: Cambridge University Press, 2021. 9781108920698 (DLC) 2020031749

Decriminalizing mental illness

LCCN	2020031749
Type of material	Book
Main title	Decriminalizing mental illness / edited by Katherine Warburton, Stephen M. Stahl.

Published/Produced	Cambridge; New York, NY: Cambridge University Press, 2021.
Description	1 online resource
ISBN	9781108920698 (ebook) (paperback)
LC classification	RA1148
Related names	Warburton, Katherine D., editor. Stahl, Stephen M., 1951- editor.
Summary	"The history of serious mental illness (SMI) is grim, from a cultural as well as a treatment perspective. The conditions of individuals with psychotic disorders have swung, like a pendulum, from institutional neglect to community neglect and back again over the past several hundred years. At the core of treatment failure is a failure in mental health policy and funding, with the result usually framed as the degree of human institutionalization in jails, prisons and asylums. In the middle of the 19th century, institutions designed to deliver moral treatment were considered the humane answer to care properly for the SMI population. By the mid- 20th century, those same, now overcrowded, institutions were blamed for the horrible conditions of mistreatment of individuals with SMI. Now, as we approach the middle of the 21st century, deinstitutionalization (the answer to the cruel asylums) is purportedly at fault for homelessness, lack of treatment, and criminalization. As the pendulum swings, we are hearing cries to "bring back" the asylums"-- Provided by publisher.
Other Subjects	Forensic Psychiatry--methods Commitment of Mentally Ill--legislation & jurisprudence Criminal Law--methods Institutionalization Psychotic Disorders--therapy Insanity Defense
Notes	Includes bibliographical references and index.

Additional formats	Print version: Decriminalizing mental illness Cambridge; New York, NY: Cambridge University Press, 2021. 9781108826952 (DLC) 2020031748

Diagnostic essentials of psychopathology: a case-based approach

LCCN	2020948976
Type of material	Book
Personal name	Hammond, Cheree, author.
Main title	Diagnostic essentials of psychopathology: a case-based approach / Cheree Hammond.
Published/Produced	Thousand Oaks, California: SAGE Publications, [2022]
Description	xix, 608 pages: illustrations; 24 cm
ISBN	9781506338101 (pbk.)
	1506338100 (pbk.)
LC classification	RC469 .H347 2022
Summary	Diagnostic Essentials of Psychopathology: A Case-Based Approach by Cheree Hammond brings together dozens of fictional cases which represent a range of human experiences, featuring people of different ages, ethnicities, genders, ability levels, and religions. Each disorder has several cases associated with it to capture the truly unique nature of working with various client intersections, and half of the cases provide the correct "answers" or diagnosis to allow students to check their understanding of this process. Some cases focus on a diagnosis, others with analysis, and others let the student practice on their own as a way to further student reflection and learning. This casebook is specifically written for disciplines that are grounded in a humanistic approach (Counseling, Social Work, Counseling Psychology). The author provides a framework for using the medical model that is presented in the DSM-5. - Provided by publisher.
Contents	Chapter 1: Making Sense of the DSM 5 - Chapter 2: Eight Steps to Diagnosis: - Chapter 3: The Justification Process - Chapter 4: Case Conceptualization and Treatment Planning - Chapter

	5: Neurodevelopmental Disorders - Chapter 6: Schizophrenia Spectrum & Other Psychotic Disorders - Chapter 7: Disorders of Mood - Chapter 8: Anxiety Disorders - Chapter 9:Obsessive Compulsive and Related Disorders - Chapter 10: Sleep-Wake Disorders - Chapter 11: Trauma and Stressor Related Disorders - Chapter 12: Dissociative Disorders - Chapter 13: Somatic Symptom & Related Disorders - Chapter 14: Feeding & Eating Disorders - Chapter 15: Sexual - Chapter 16: Disruptive - Chapter 17: Substance Use Disorders - Chapter 18: Personality - Chapter 19: Paraphilic Disorders - Chapter 20: File Length Cases
LC Subjects	Psychology, Pathological--Diagnosis.
Other Subjects	Mental Disorders--diagnosis
	Psychology, Pathological--Diagnosis.
Notes	Includes bibliographical references and index.
Additional formats	ebook version: 9781506338125

Dimensions of psychological problems: replacing diagnostic categories with a more science-based and less stigmatizing alternative

LCCN	2021015168
Type of material	Book
Personal name	Lahey, Benjamin B., author.
Main title	Dimensions of psychological problems: replacing diagnostic categories with a more science-based and less stigmatizing alternative / Benjamin B. Lahey.
Published/Produced	New York, NY: Oxford University Press, [2021]
Description	1 online resource
ISBN	9780197607923 (epub)
	9780197607930 (online)
	(paperback)
LC classification	RC454
Summary	"Psychological problems are simply aspects of our behavior- broadly defined to include our ways of thinking, perceiving, feeling, and acting-that cause us distress or interfere with functioning in important areas of our lives. This straightforward and pragmatic definition of psychological problems is offered as an

Bibliography

alternative to the current medical model view in the Diagnostic and Statistical Manual of Mental Disorders published by the American Psychiatric Association and the International Classification of Diseases published by the World Health Organization that dominates thinking about psychological problems in most of the world today. Psychological problems are not the result of terrifying illnesses of the mind. Although can be very distressing and problematic for individuals, they are surprisingly commonplace variations in the natural continua of psychological problems that arise in perfectly ordinary ways. This perspective has the advantages of scientific validity and reducing the stigma inherent in viewing psychological problems as mental illnesses, mental disorders, or psychopathology"-- Provided by publisher.

Contents — Conceptualizing psychological problems - From binary diagnostic categories to dimensions of psychological problems - Dimensions of internalizing problems - Dimensions of externalizing problems - Dimensions of psychotic and other problems of thought and affect - Hierarchical nature of psychological problems - Sex differences and the development of psychological problems - Ordinary origins of psychological problems: gene-environment interplay - Ordinary origins of psychological problems: transacting with the world.

Other Subjects — Diagnostic and statistical manual of mental disorders. 5th ed.
Mental Disorders--etiology
Adaptation, Psychological
International Classification of Diseases
Social Factors

Notes — Includes bibliographical references and index.

Additional formats — Print version: Lahey, Benjamin B. Dimensions of psychological problems New York, NY: Oxford University Press, [2021] 9780197607909 (DLC) 2021015167

Dimensions of psychological problems: replacing diagnostic categories with a more science-based and less stigmatizing alternative

LCCN	2021015167
Type of material	Book
Personal name	Lahey, Benjamin B., author.
Main title	Dimensions of psychological problems: replacing diagnostic categories with a more science-based and less stigmatizing alternative / Benjamin B. Lahey.
Published/Produced	New York, NY: Oxford University Press, [2021]
ISBN	9780197607909 (paperback) (epub) (online)
LC classification	RC454
Summary	"Psychological problems are simply aspects of our behavior- broadly defined to include our ways of thinking, perceiving, feeling, and acting-that cause us distress or interfere with functioning in important areas of our lives. This straightforward and pragmatic definition of psychological problems is offered as an alternative to the current medical model view in the Diagnostic and Statistical Manual of Mental Disorders published by the American Psychiatric Association and the International Classification of Diseases published by the World Health Organization that dominates thinking about psychological problems in most of the world today. Psychological problems are not the result of terrifying illnesses of the mind. Although can be very distressing and problematic for individuals, they are surprisingly commonplace variations in the natural continua of psychological problems that arise in perfectly ordinary ways. This perspective has the advantages of scientific validity and reducing the stigma inherent in viewing psychological problems as mental illnesses, mental disorders, or psychopathology"-- Provided by publisher.
Contents	Conceptualizing psychological problems - From binary diagnostic categories to dimensions of psychological problems - Dimensions of

	internalizing problems - Dimensions of externalizing problems - Dimensions of psychotic and other problems of thought and affect - Hierarchical nature of psychological problems - Sex differences and the development of psychological problems - Ordinary origins of psychological problems: gene-environment interplay - Ordinary origins of psychological problems: transacting with the world.
Other Subjects	Diagnostic and statistical manual of mental disorders. 5th ed.
	Mental Disorders--etiology
	Adaptation, Psychological
	International Classification of Diseases
	Social Factors
Notes	Includes bibliographical references and index.
Additional formats	Online version: Lahey, Benjamin B., Dimensions of psychological problems New York, NY: Oxford University Press, [2021] 9780197607923 (DLC) 2021015168

First aid for the psychiatry clerkship

LCCN	2021004054
Type of material	Book
Personal name	Ganti, Latha, author.
Main title	First aid for the psychiatry clerkship / Sean M. Blitzstein, Lantha Ganti, Matthew S. Kaufman.
Edition	Sixth edition.
Published/Produced	New York: McGraw Hill, [2021]
ISBN	9781264257843 (paperback; alk. paper)
	1264257848 (paperback; alk. paper)
	(ebook)
	(ebook)
LC classification	RC454
Related names	Kaufman, Matthew S., author.
	Blitzstein, Sean, author.
Summary	"Each of the chapters in this book contains the major topics central to the practice of psychiatry and has been specifically designed for the medical student learning level, to excel in the clerkship (shelf exams),

Contents	as well as the USMLE Step 2 and 3 exams"-- Provided by publisher. How to succeed in the psychiatry clerkship - Examination and diagnosis - Psychotic disorders - Mood disorders - Anxiety, obsessive-compulsive, trauma, and stressor-related disorders - Personality disorders - Substance-related and addictive disorders - Neurocognitive disorders - Geriatric psychiatry - Psychiatric disorders in children - Dissociative disorders - Somatic symptom and factitious disorders - Impulse control disorders - Eating disorders - Sleep-wake disorders - Sexual dysfunctions and paraphilic disorders - Psychotherapies - Psychopharmacology - Forensic psychiatry.
Other Subjects	Mental Disorders Clinical Clerkship Psychiatry
Form/Genre	Outline
Notes	Includes index.
Additional formats	Online version: Ganti, Latha. First aid for the psychiatry clerkship. Sixth edition New York: McGraw Hill, [2021] 9781264257850 (DLC) 2021004055

First aid for the psychiatry clerkship

LCCN	2021004055
Type of material	Book
Personal name	Ganti, Latha, author.
Main title	First aid for the psychiatry clerkship / Sean M. Blitzstein, Lantha Ganti, Matthew S. Kaufman.
Edition	Sixth edition.
Published/Produced	New York: McGraw Hill, [2021]
Description	1 online resource
ISBN	1264257856 (ebook) 9781264257850 (ebook) (paperback; alk. paper) (paperback; alk. paper)
LC classification	RC454

Bibliography

Related names	Kaufman, Matthew S., author.
	Blitzstein, Sean, author.
Summary	"Each of the chapters in this book contains the major topics central to the practice of psychiatry and has been specifically designed for the medical student learning level, to excel in the clerkship (shelf exams), as well as the USMLE Step 2 and 3 exams"-- Provided by publisher.
Contents	How to succeed in the psychiatry clerkship - Examination and diagnosis - Psychotic disorders - Mood disorders - Anxiety, obsessive-compulsive, trauma, and stressor-related disorders - Personality disorders - Substance-related and addictive disorders - Neurocognitive disorders - Geriatric psychiatry - Psychiatric disorders in children - Dissociative disorders - Somatic symptom and factitious disorders - Impulse control disorders - Eating disorders - Sleep-wake disorders - Sexual dysfunctions and paraphilic disorders - Psychotherapies - Psychopharmacology - Forensic psychiatry.
Other Subjects	Mental Disorders
	Clinical Clerkship
	Psychiatry
Form/Genre	Outline
Notes	Includes index.
Additional formats	Print version: Ganti, Latha. First aid for the psychiatry clerkship. Sixth edition New York: McGraw Hill, [2021] 9781264257843 (DLC) 2021004054

Handbook of geropsychiatry for the advanced practice nurse: mental healthcare for the older adult

LCCN	2020052122
Type of material	Book
Main title	Handbook of geropsychiatry for the advanced practice nurse: mental healthcare for the older adult / Leigh Powers, Marie Smith-East, editors.
Published/Produced	New York: Springer Publishing Company, [2021]
Description	1 online resource

ISBN	9780826157515 (ebook) (paperback)
LC classification	RC954
Related names	Powers, Leigh, DNP, editor. Smith-East, Marie, editor.
Summary	"The ability to reduce the burden of illness among older adults is necessary as individuals are living longer and experiencing lower rates of disability (National Institute on Aging, 2020). Advanced practice nurses are skilled to relieve the burden of illness among older adults through specialized training and providing treatment in a variety of clinical settings. While geriatric-focused content exists, advanced practice nurses can benefit from clinical pearls specific for the advanced practice nurse providing holistic mental healthcare"-- Provided by publisher.
Contents	Basic foundations of aging / Leigh Powers - The psychiatric exam in geropsychiatry / Leigh Powers - Depressive disorders / Deana Goldin - Bipolar and related disorders / Dr. Helene Vossos - Anxiety disorders / Abimbola Farinde, Leigh Powers, Marie Smith-East - Schizophrenia spectrum and other psychotic disorders / Marie Smith-East - Sleep-wake disorders / Leigh Powers - Substance-related and addictive disorders / Dr. Helene Vossos, David J. Mokler, Marie Smith-East - Neurocognitive disorders / William Sutton - Sexual dysfunction in geropsychiatry / Matthew Keeslar, Alan W. Skipper, Joanne Zanetos - Medication issues and prescribing in geropsychiatry / David J. Mokler, Marie Smith-East - Elder Abuse / Marie Smith-East - Family dynamics / Marie Smith-East - Palliative care and end of life issues / Marie Smith-East - Caring for patients during a pandemic / Marie Smith-East.
Other Subjects	Mental Disorders--nursing Geriatric Nursing--methods Advanced Practice Nursing--methods Aged--psychology

	Nursing Assessment--methods
Notes	Includes bibliographical references and index.
Additional formats	Print version: Handbook of geropsychiatry for the advanced practice nurse New York: Springer Publishing Company, [2021] 9780826157492 (DLC) 2020052121

How madness shaped history: an eccentric array of maniacal rulers, raving narcissists, and psychotic visionaries

LCCN	2019980937
Type of material	Book
Personal name	Ferguson, Christopher J., author.
Main title	How madness shaped history: an eccentric array of maniacal rulers, raving narcissists, and psychotic visionaries / Christopher Ferguson.
Published/Produced	Amherst: Prometheus Books, 2020.
Description	1 online resource
ISBN	9781633885752 (ebook)
	(hardcover)
LC classification	RC438
Summary	"This book considers the impact of psychology on world events, looking at how mental illness and personality disorders have affected history"-- Provided by publisher.
LC Subjects	Mental illness--History.
	Psychoses--History.
Notes	Includes bibliographical references and index.
Additional formats	Print version: Ferguson, Christopher J.. How madness shaped history Amherst: Prometheus Books, 2020. 9781633885745 (DLC) 2019020144

How madness shaped history: an eccentric array of maniacal rulers, raving narcissists, and psychotic visionaries

LCCN	2019020144
Type of material	Book
Personal name	Ferguson, Christopher J., author.
Main title	How madness shaped history: an eccentric array of maniacal rulers, raving narcissists, and psychotic visionaries / Christopher Ferguson.

Published/Produced	Amherst: Prometheus Books, 2020.
Description	295 pages; 24 cm
ISBN	9781633885745 (hardcover)
	(ebook)
LC classification	RC438, F47 2020
Summary	"This book considers the impact of psychology on world events, looking at how mental illness and personality disorders have affected history"-- Provided by publisher.
LC Subjects	Mental illness--History.
	Psychoses--History.
Notes	Includes bibliographical references and index.
Additional formats	Online version: Ferguson, Christopher J., How madness shaped history Amherst: 2020. 9781633885752 (DLC) 2019980937

Immunopsychiatry: an introduction

LCCN	2021024612
Type of material	Book
Uniform title	Immunopsychiatry (Khandaker)
Main title	Immunopsychiatry: an introduction / edited by Golam Khandaker, Neil Harrison, Edward Bullmore, Robert Dantzer.
Published/Produced	Cambridge, United Kingdom; New York, NY: Cambridge University Press, 2021.
ISBN	9781108424042 (hardback)
	(ebook)
LC classification	RC454
Related names	Khandaker, Golam M., editor.
	Harrison, Neil (Neil Andrew), editor.
	Bullmore, Edward T., editor.
	Dantzer, Robert, editor.
Summary	"Once thought to be an immune-privileged site, we now know that there is a complex and essential bidirectional interplay between the central nervous system (CNS) and the immune system. Technological advances in imaging, genomic medicine and immunology have resulted in major revisions to some of the most fundamental and long-

held assumptions in neuroscience, and we now understand that the immune system is critically involved not only in brain pathology, but also in the normal processes of brain development and homeostasis. 'Immunopsychiatry', namely the study of the interactions between neuroscience, mental health and the immune system, has rapidly become a major priority for psychiatric research. Accumulating evidence indicates roles for the immune system in the pathophysiology of many neurodegenerative and psychiatric disorders including Alzheimer's disease (AD), schizophrenia, major depressive disorder (MDD), multiple sclerosis (MS) and others. In particular, pro-inflammatory cytokines associated with inflammation, which is common to many of these disorders, can influence the brain to bring about a host of physiological as well as behavioural alterations such as changes in mood and cognition. Raised pro-inflammatory cytokines are consistently reported in MDD and schizophrenia. Moreover, systemic inflammation brought about by acute infection, diabetes, obesity and atherosclerosis can accelerate cognitive decline in the elderly and present significant risk for the development or acceleration of AD and delirium. With this new knowledge come new targets to be exploited as biomarkers for diagnosis or informing treatment. A number of immunemodulating therapeutics are currently being trialled for the treatment of MDD, schizophrenia, AD and others"-- Provided by publisher.

Contents Basic concepts in immunobiology / Lorinda Turner and Neil Harrison - The evolution of immunological research in psychiatric disorders / Prof Keith Kelley - Stress, immune system and the brain / Julie-Myrtille Bourgognon, Alison McColl, Maria Suessmilch, Rajeev Krishnadas and Jonathan Cavanagh - Role of infection and inflammatory cytokines / Prof Alan Brown, Fiona Conway, Genvieive Falabella and Carly Apar - Role of auto-immunity, anti-NMDA

	receptor and related antibodies / Mike Zandi and Esha Abrol - Effectiveness of Immunotherapies for Psychotic Disorders / Rachel Upthegrove and Bill Deakin - Inflammation, sickness behaviour and depression / Neil Harrison, Alessandro Colasanti and Golam Khandaker - Inflammation, antidepressant response and immunotherapies for depression / Golam Khandaker, Prof Ed Bullmore and Nils Kappelmann - Role of Microglia in Neurodegenerative Disease / Colm Cunningham and Donal Skelly - Role of inflammation in Parkinson's disease dementia and dementia with Lewy body / John O'Brien and Ajenthan Surendranathan - The role of adaptive and innate immunity in Alzheimer's disease / Clive Holmes - The immune system and anxiety disorders / Vasaliki Michopoulos and Tanja Jovanovic - Microbiome-gut-brain interactions in autism and other neurodevelopmental disorders / John Cryan, Ted Dinan, Kiran Sandhu and Eoin Sherwin - Role of the adaptive immune system in resolution of inflammation-associated disorders / Prof Robert Dantzer - Trans-diagnostic effect of immune system on psychiatric disorders / Prof Bernhard T. Baune.
Other Subjects	Mental Disorders--Immunology. Immune System--Immunology. Immunotherapy--methods Medical / Mental Health Medical / Mental Health
Notes	Includes bibliographical references and index.
Additional formats	Online version: Immunopsychiatry Cambridge, United Kingdom; New York, NY: Cambridge University Press, 2021 9781108539623 (DLC) 2021024613

Immunopsychiatry: an introduction

LCCN	2021024613
Type of material	Book
Uniform title	Immunopsychiatry (Khandaker)

Main title	Immunopsychiatry: an introduction / edited by Golam Khandaker, Neil Harrison, Edward Bullmore, Robert Dantzer.
Published/Produced	Cambridge, United Kingdom; New York, NY: Cambridge University Press, 2021.
Description	1 online resource
ISBN	9781108539623 (ebook) (hardback)
LC classification	RC454
Related names	Khandaker, Golam M., editor. Harrison, Neil (Neil Andrew), editor. Bullmore, Edward T., editor. Dantzer, Robert, editor.
Summary	"Once thought to be an immune-privileged site, we now know that there is a complex and essential bidirectional interplay between the central nervous system (CNS) and the immune system. Technological advances in imaging, genomic medicine and immunology have resulted in major revisions to some of the most fundamental and long-held assumptions in neuroscience, and we now understand that the immune system is critically involved not only in brain pathology, but also in the normal processes of brain development and homeostasis. 'Immunopsychiatry', namely the study of the interactions between neuroscience, mental health and the immune system, has rapidly become a major priority for psychiatric research. Accumulating evidence indicates roles for the immune system in the pathophysiology of many neurodegenerative and psychiatric disorders including Alzheimer's disease (AD), schizophrenia, major depressive disorder (MDD), multiple sclerosis (MS) and others. In particular, pro-inflammatory cytokines associated with inflammation, which is common to many of these disorders, can influence the brain to bring about a host of physiological as well as behavioural alterations such as changes in mood and cognition. Raised pro-inflammatory cytokines are consistently

reported in MDD and schizophrenia. Moreover, systemic inflammation brought about by acute infection, diabetes, obesity and atherosclerosis can accelerate cognitive decline in the elderly and present significant risk for the development or acceleration of AD and delirium. With this new knowledge come new targets to be exploited as biomarkers for diagnosis or informing treatment. A number of immunemodulating therapeutics are currently being trialled for the treatment of MDD, schizophrenia, AD and others"-- Provided by publisher.

Contents Basic concepts in immunobiology / Lorinda Turner and Neil Harrison - The evolution of immunological research in psychiatric disorders / Prof Keith Kelley - Stress, immune system and the brain / Julie-Myrtille Bourgognon, Alison McColl, Maria Suessmilch, Rajeev Krishnadas and Jonathan Cavanagh - Role of infection and inflammatory cytokines / Prof Alan Brown, Fiona Conway, Genvieive Falabella and Carly Apar - Role of auto-immunity, anti-NMDA receptor and related antibodies / Mike Zandi and Esha Abrol - Effectiveness of Immunotherapies for Psychotic Disorders / Rachel Upthegrove and Bill Deakin - Inflammation, sickness behaviour and depression / Neil Harrison, Alessandro Colasanti and Golam Khandaker - Inflammation, antidepressant response and immunotherapies for depression / Golam Khandaker, Prof Ed Bullmore and Nils Kappelmann - Role of Microglia in Neurodegenerative Disease / Colm Cunningham and Donal Skelly - Role of inflammation in Parkinson's disease dementia and dementia with Lewy body / John O'Brien and Ajenthan Surendranathan - The role of adaptive and innate immunity in Alzheimer's disease / Clive Holmes - The immune system and anxiety disorders / Vasaliki Michopoulos and Tanja Jovanovic - Microbiome-gut-brain interactions in autism and other neurodevelopmental disorders / John Cryan, Ted Dinan, Kiran Sandhu and Eoin

	Sherwin - Role of the adaptive immune system in resolution of inflammation-associated disorders / Prof Robert Dantzer - Trans-diagnostic effect of immune system on psychiatric disorders / Prof Bernhard T. Baune.
Other Subjects	Mental Disorders--Immunology.
	Immune System--Immunology.
	Immunotherapy--methods
	Medical / Mental Health
	Medical / Mental Health
Notes	Includes bibliographical references and index.
Additional formats	Print version: Immunopsychiatry (Khandaker) Immunopsychiatry Cambridge, United Kingdom; New York, NY: Cambridge University Press, 2021 9781108424042 (DLC) 2021024612

Integrative group therapy for psychosis: an evidence-based approach

LCCN	2020013790
Type of material	Book
Personal name	Kanas, Nick, 1945- author.
Main title	Integrative group therapy for psychosis: an evidence-based approach / Nick Kanas.
Published/Produced	New York, NY: Routledge/Taylor & Francis Group, 2021.
Description	1 online resource
ISBN	9781003056553 (ebook)
	(hardback)
	(paperback)
LC classification	RC454
Summary	"Through a series of outcome and process studies, this book presents an evidence-based integrative treatment model that includes elements from psychodynamic, interpersonal, psychoeducational, and cognitive-behavioral therapy (CBT) approaches to address the needs of people suffering from psychosis. Designed to help patients deal with delusions, hallucinations, disorganized thinking, interpersonal problems, and the stigma of having a serious mental illness, the book chronicles the

	evolution of the integrative approach from clinical research in inpatient and outpatient settings to theoretical and clinical issues that were derived from the empirical studies. Chapters also include information and vignettes to assist the reader on in conducting therapy groups for patients suffering from acute and chronic psychosis. Shown to be a safe and supportive adjunct to medications that is useful in both inpatient and outpatient settings, readers will find value in this unique, empirically-driven model for groups that are long-term, short-term, and time-limited"-- Provided by publisher.
Contents	Nature of psychotic conditions - Historical and clinical issues - Research issues - Clinical issues of the integrative model: the basics - Clinical issues of the integrative model: special topics - Evaluation of the integrative model - Integrative groups for non-psychotic bipolar patients.
Other Subjects	Psychotic Disorders--therapy Psychotherapy, Group--methods Integrative Medicine Evidence-Based Medicine
Notes	Includes bibliographical references and index.
Additional formats	Print version: Kanas, Nick, 1945- Integrative group therapy for psychosis New York, NY: Routledge/ Taylor & Francis Group, 2021 9780367340391 (DLC) 2020013789

Integrative group therapy for psychosis: an evidence-based approach

LCCN	2020013789
Type of material	Book
Personal name	Kanas, Nick, 1945- author.
Main title	Integrative group therapy for psychosis: an evidence-based approach / Nick Kanas.
Published/Produced	New York, NY: Routledge, 2021.
ISBN	9780367340391 (hardback) 9780367339425 (paperback) (ebook)
LC classification	RC454

Bibliography

Summary	"Through a series of outcome and process studies, this book presents an evidence-based integrative treatment model that includes elements from psychodynamic, interpersonal, psychoeducational, and cognitive-behavioral therapy (CBT) approaches to address the needs of people suffering from psychosis. Designed to help patients deal with delusions, hallucinations, disorganized thinking, interpersonal problems, and the stigma of having a serious mental illness, the book chronicles the evolution of the integrative approach from clinical research in inpatient and outpatient settings to theoretical and clinical issues that were derived from the empirical studies. Chapters also include information and vignettes to assist the reader on in conducting therapy groups for patients suffering from acute and chronic psychosis. Shown to be a safe and supportive adjunct to medications that is useful in both inpatient and outpatient settings, readers will find value in this unique, empirically-driven model for groups that are long-term, short-term, and time-limited"-- Provided by publisher.
Contents	Nature of psychotic conditions - Historical and clinical issues - Research issues - Clinical issues of the integrative model: the basics - Clinical issues of the integrative model: special topics - Evaluation of the integrative model - Integrative groups for non-psychotic bipolar patients.
Other Subjects	Psychotic Disorders--therapy Psychotherapy, Group--methods Integrative Medicine Evidence-Based Medicine
Notes	Includes bibliographical references and index.
Additional formats	Online version: Kanas, Nick, 1945- Integrative group therapy for psychosis New York, NY: Routledge/ Taylor & Francis Group, 2021 9781003056553 (DLC) 2020013790

Introductory textbook of psychiatry

LCCN	2020008707
Type of material	Book
Personal name	Black, Donald W., 1956- author.
Main title	Introductory textbook of psychiatry / Donald W. Black, M.D., Nancy C. Andreasen, M.D., Ph.D.
Edition	Seventh edition.
Published/Produced	Washington, DC: American Psychiatric Association Publishing, [2021]
Description	xvii, 619 pages: illustrations; 23 cm
ISBN	9781615373123 (hardcover; alk. paper)
	9781615373192 (paperback)
	(ebook)
LC classification	RC454 .A427 2021
Related names	Andreasen, Nancy C., author.
	American Psychiatric Association, issuing body.
Summary	"The Introductory Textbook of Psychiatry provides a comprehensive introduction to the field both for students new to psychiatry and for students who are studying for their board exams. This authoritative, seventh edition has been thoroughly updated to reflect advances since the last edition. DSM-5® provides a frame for the text's many illuminating clinical vignettes, which in turn bring diagnosis, assessment, and treatment to vivid life. Other features, such as clinical points, self-assessment questions, and an exhaustive glossary of terms, add to the educational value and enhance learning. The internationally renowned authors have produced a text of uniform approach and uncommon style, and readers will appreciate the insight and rigor that have made the Introductory Textbook of Psychiatry the bestselling volume of its kind for more than two decades"-- Provided by publisher.
Contents	Diagnosis and Classification - Interviewing and Assessment - Neurobiology and Genetics of Mental Illness - Neurodevelopmental (Child) Disorders - Schizophrenia Spectrum and Other Psychotic Disorders - Mood Disorders - Anxiety Disorders -

	Obsessive-Compulsive and Related Disorders - Trauma- and Stressor-Related Disorders - Somatic Symptom Disorders and Dissociative Disorders - Feeding and Eating Disorders - Sleep-Wake Disorders - Sexual Dysfunction, Gender Dysphoria, and Paraphilic Disorders - Disruptive, Impulse-Control, and Conduct Disorders - Substance-Related and Addictive Disorders - Neurocognitive Disorders. - Personality Disorders - Psychiatric Emergencies - Legal Issues - Psychotherapy - Somatic Treatments.
Other Subjects	Mental Disorders
	Psychiatry--methods
Notes	Includes bibliographical references and index.
Additional formats	Online version: Black, Donald W., 1956- Introductory textbook of psychiatry Seventh edition. Arlington, VA: American Psychiatric Association Publishing, [2021] 9781615373185 (DLC) 2020008708

Introductory textbook of psychiatry

LCCN	2020008708
Type of material	Book
Personal name	Black, Donald W., 1956 author.
Main title	Introductory textbook of psychiatry / Donald W. Black, Nancy C. Andreasen.
Edition	Seventh edition.
Published/Produced	Arlington, VA: American Psychiatric Association Publishing, [2021]
Description	1 online resource
ISBN	9781615373185 (ebook)
	(hardcover; alk. paper)
	(paperback)
LC classification	RC454
Related names	Andreasen, Nancy C., author.
	American Psychiatric Association, issuing body.
Summary	"The Introductory Textbook of Psychiatry provides a comprehensive introduction to the field both for students new to psychiatry and for students who are studying for their board exams. This authoritative,

Bibliography

	seventh edition has been thoroughly updated to reflect advances since the last edition. DSM-5® provides a frame for the text's many illuminating clinical vignettes, which in turn bring diagnosis, assessment, and treatment to vivid life. Other features, such as clinical points, self-assessment questions, and an exhaustive glossary of terms, add to the educational value and enhance learning. The internationally renowned authors have produced a text of uniform approach and uncommon style, and readers will appreciate the insight and rigor that have made the Introductory Textbook of Psychiatry the bestselling volume of its kind for more than two decades"-- Provided by publisher.
Contents	Diagnosis and Classification - Interviewing and Assessment - Neurobiology and Genetics of Mental Illness - Neurodevelopmental (Child) Disorders - Schizophrenia Spectrum and Other Psychotic Disorders - Mood Disorders - Anxiety Disorders - Obsessive-Compulsive and Related Disorders - Trauma- and Stressor-Related Disorders - Somatic Symptom Disorders and Dissociative Disorders - Feeding and Eating Disorders - Sleep-Wake Disorders - Sexual Dysfunction, Gender Dysphoria, and Paraphilic Disorders - Disruptive, Impulse-Control, and Conduct Disorders - Substance-Related and Addictive Disorders - Neurocognitive Disorders. - Personality Disorders - Psychiatric Emergencies - Legal Issues - Psychotherapy - Somatic Treatments.
Other Subjects	Mental Disorders
	Psychiatry--methods
Notes	Includes bibliographical references and index.
Additional formats	Print version: Black, Donald W., 1956- Introductory textbook of psychiatry Seventh edition. Arlington, VA: American Psychiatric Association Publishing, [2021] 9781615373123 (DLC) 2020008707

Bibliography

Let's talk about religion and mental health

LCCN	2021016453
Type of material	Book
Personal name	Judd, Daniel K, author.
Main title	Let's talk about religion and mental health / Daniel K Judd.
Published/Produced	Salt Lake City, Utah: Deseret Book, [2021] ©2021
ISBN	9781629728254 (paperback)
LC classification	BX8643.M45 J83 2021
Summary	"Latter-day Saint author Daniel K Judd discusses mental health in the context of believing Latter-day Saint doctrine and policy"-- Provided by publisher.
Contents	Depression, sickness, sorrow, and the gospel of Jesus Christ - Anxiety and the grace of Jesus Christ - Psychotic disorders, self-deception and divine revelation - Parents, children, and mental health - Healing the broken brain - Healing the broken heart.
LC Subjects	Mental health--Religious aspects--Church of Jesus Christ of Latter-day Saints. Mental health--Religious aspects--Mormon Church. Mormons--Mental health.
Notes	Includes bibliographical references and index.
Series	Let's talk about

Management of complex treatment-resistant psychotic disorders

LCCN	2020055182
Type of material	Book
Main title	Management of complex treatment-resistant psychotic disorders / edited by Dr. Michael A. Cummings, Dr. Stephen M. Stahl.
Published/Produced	Cambridge, United Kingdom; New York: Cambridge University Press, 2021.
Description	1 online resource
ISBN	9781108963923 (ebook) (paperback)
LC classification	RM333.5
Related names	Cummings, Michael A. (Michael Allen), 1951- editor.

Summary	Stahl, Stephen M., 1951- editor. "In community settings, the most common barriers to independent living, employment, and stable interpersonal relationships for patients suffering from schizophrenia-spectrum disorders or other psychotic disorders are negative symptoms and cognitive deficits. In contrast, severely mentally ill individuals, often incarcerated or chronically institutionalized, more frequently experience substantial barriers related to positive psychotic symptoms leading to problematic behaviors such as aggression or violence. This is not to say that among the chronically institutionalized severely mentally ill population that positive psychotic symptoms are the only, or even majority, source of problematic behaviors. A survey conducted within the California Department of State Hospitals, a circa 7000-bed system dedicated to the treatment of conserved and forensically committed patients, reviewed 839 episodes of aggression or violence by 88 persistently aggressive inpatients and found that 54% of such episodes were impulsive, 39% were predatory or instrumental, and 17% were psychotically driven. Nevertheless, amelioration or control of positive psychotic symptoms commonly forms the initial treatment focus among the severely mentally ill."-- Provided by publisher.
Other Subjects	Psychotic Disorders--drug therapy Psychotic Disorders--complications Antipsychotic Agents--therapeutic use Antipsychotic Agents--pharmacology Psychopharmacology--methods Drug Resistance
Notes	Includes bibliographical references and index.
Additional formats	Print version: Management of complex treatment-resistant psychotic disorders Cambridge, United Kingdom; New York: Cambridge University Press, 2021. 9781108965682 (DLC) 2020055181

Management of complex treatment-resistant psychotic disorders

LCCN	2020055181
Type of material	Book
Main title	Management of complex treatment-resistant psychotic disorders / edited by Dr. Michael A. Cummings, Dr. Stephen M. Stahl.
Published/Produced	Cambridge, United Kingdom; New York: Cambridge University Press, 2021.
ISBN	9781108965682 (paperback) (ebook)
LC classification	RM333.5
Related names	Cummings, Michael A. (Michael Allen), 1951- editor.
	Stahl, Stephen M., 1951- editor.
Summary	"In community settings, the most common barriers to independent living, employment, and stable interpersonal relationships for patients suffering from schizophrenia-spectrum disorders or other psychotic disorders are negative symptoms and cognitive deficits. In contrast, severely mentally ill individuals, often incarcerated or chronically institutionalized, more frequently experience substantial barriers related to positive psychotic symptoms leading to problematic behaviors such as aggression or violence. This is not to say that among the chronically institutionalized severely mentally ill population that positive psychotic symptoms are the only, or even majority, source of problematic behaviors. A survey conducted within the California Department of State Hospitals, a circa 7000-bed system dedicated to the treatment of conserved and forensically committed patients, reviewed 839 episodes of aggression or violence by 88 persistently aggressive inpatients and found that 54% of such episodes were impulsive, 39% were predatory or instrumental, and 17% were psychotically driven. Nevertheless, amelioration or control of positive psychotic symptoms commonly forms the initial treatment focus among the severely mentally ill."-- Provided by publisher.

Other Subjects	Psychotic Disorders--drug therapy
	Psychotic Disorders--complications
	Antipsychotic Agents--therapeutic use
	Antipsychotic Agents--pharmacology
	Psychopharmacology--methods
	Drug Resistance
Notes	Includes bibliographical references and index.
Additional formats	Online version: Management of complex treatment-resistant psychotic disorders Cambridge, United Kingdom; New York: Cambridge University Press, 2021. 9781108963923 (DLC) 2020055182

Management of sleep disorders in psychiatry

LCCN	2019040663
Type of material	Book
Main title	Management of sleep disorders in psychiatry / [edited by] Amit Chopra, Piyush Das, Karl Doghramji.
Published/Produced	New York, NY: Oxford University Press, [2020]
ISBN	9780190929671 (hb)
	(epub)
	(updf)
LC classification	RC547
Related names	Chopra, Amit, editor.
	Das, Piyush, MD, editor.
	Doghramji, Karl, editor.
Summary	"Virtually every biological function in humans depends on normal sleep homeostasis to maintain normalcy. As will be evidenced throughout this volume, sleep and its disturbance are intimately linked to normal brain function and psychiatric disorders, respectively"-- Provided by publisher.
Contents	Sleep Medicine and Psychiatry: The Inseparable Two - Sleep Architecture and Physiology - Neurobiology of Sleep and Wakefulness - Circadian rhythms - Sleep and Cognition - Office based Evaluation of Sleep Disordered Patients - Clinical Applications of Technical Procedures in Sleep Medicine - Insomnia disorder-Pathophysiology - Insomnia disorder: Pharmacological treatments - Insomnia disorder:

	Behavioral Treatments - Hypersomnolence disorders - Parasomnias - Circadian rhythm Sleep-Wake disorders - Sleep-Related Movement Disorders - Breathing-Related Sleep Disorders - Pediatric sleep-wake disorders - Depressive Disorders - Bipolar and Related Disorders - Anxiety Disorders - Trauma and Stressor-Related disorders: Schizophrenia Spectrum and Other Psychotic disorders - Substance-Related and Addictive Disorders - Neurodevelopmental disorders - Delirium - Neurocognitive Disorders - Neuropsychiatric disorders - Pain Disorders - Psychotropic medications and Sleep - Forensic Sleep Medicine - Eating Disorders - Future of Sleep Medicine and Psychiatry
Other Subjects	Sleep Wake Disorders--therapy Psychiatry--methods
Notes	Includes bibliographical references and index.
Additional formats	Online version: Chopra, Amit, Management of sleep disorders in psychiatry New York: Oxford University Press, 2020. 9780190929695 (DLC) 2019040664

Management of sleep disorders in psychiatry

LCCN	2019040664
Type of material	Book
Main title	Management of sleep disorders in psychiatry / [edited by] Amit Chopra, Piyush Das, Karl Doghramji.
Published/Produced	New York, NY: Oxford University Press, [2020]
Description	1 online resource
ISBN	9780190929688 (updf) 9780190929695 (epub) (hb)
LC classification	RC547
Related names	Chopra, Amit, editor. Das, Piyush, MD, editor. Doghramji, Karl, editor.
Summary	"Virtually every biological function in humans depends on normal sleep homeostasis to maintain normalcy. As will be evidenced throughout this volume, sleep and its disturbance are intimately

Contents	linked to normal brain function and psychiatric disorders, respectively"-- Provided by publisher. Sleep Medicine and Psychiatry: The Inseparable Two - Sleep Architecture and Physiology - Neurobiology of Sleep and Wakefulness - Circadian rhythms - Sleep and Cognition - Office based Evaluation of Sleep Disordered Patients - Clinical Applications of Technical Procedures in Sleep Medicine - Insomnia disorder-Pathophysiology - Insomnia disorder: Pharmacological treatments - Insomnia disorder: Behavioral Treatments - Hypersomnolence disorders - Parasomnias - Circadian rhythm Sleep-Wake disorders - Sleep-Related Movement Disorders - Breathing-Related Sleep Disorders - Pediatric sleep-wake disorders - Depressive Disorders - Bipolar and Related Disorders - Anxiety Disorders - Trauma and Stressor-Related disorders: Schizophrenia Spectrum and Other Psychotic disorders - Substance-Related and Addictive Disorders - Neurodevelopmental disorders - Delirium - Neurocognitive Disorders - Neuropsychiatric disorders - Pain Disorders - Psychotropic medications and Sleep - Forensic Sleep Medicine - Eating Disorders - Future of Sleep Medicine and Psychiatry
Other Subjects	Sleep Wake Disorders--therapy Psychiatry--methods
Notes	Includes bibliographical references and index.
Additional formats	Print version: Management of sleep disorders in psychiatry New York, NY: Oxford University Press, [2020] 9780190929671 (DLC) 2019040663

Mental health disorders on television: representation versus reality

LCCN	2020015191
Type of material	Book
Personal name	McMahon-Coleman, Kimberley, author.
Main title	Mental health disorders on television: representation versus reality / Kimberley McMahon-Coleman and Roslyn Weaver.

Published/Produced	Jefferson, North Carolina: McFarland & Company, Inc., Publishers, [2020]
Description	ix, 173 pages; 23 cm
ISBN	9781476672151 (print) (ebook)
LC classification	PN1992.8.M46 M37 2020
Related names	Weaver, Roslyn, 1979- author.
Summary	""In past decades portrayals of mental illness on television were limited to psychotic criminals or comical sidekicks. As public awareness of mental illness has increased so too have its depictions on the small screen. A gradual transition from stereotypes towards more nuanced representations has seen a wide range of lead characters with mental health disorders, including schizophrenia, bipolar disorder, OCD, autism spectrum disorder, dissociative identity disorder, anxiety, depression and PTSD. But what are these portrayals saying about mental health and how closely do they align with real-life experiences? Drawing on interviews with people living with mental illness, this book traces these shifts, placing on-screen depictions in context and demonstrating their real world impacts."-- Provided by publisher.
Contents	Acknowledgments - Preface - Introduction - One. "I don't pick up on signs": Autism Spectrum Disorder - Two. "It's a gift and a curse": Obsessive Compulsive Disorder - Three. "Tell me who I am": Schizophrenia and Dissociative Identity Disorder - Four. "The inspirational, the enthusiastic, the unusual": Bipolar Disorder - Five. "Maybe I don't have the right genetic make up": Depression, Anxiety and Post-Traumatic Stress Disorder - Six. "The reality is much murkier": Reality and Representation - Conclusion - References - Index.
LC Subjects	Mental illness on television.
Notes	Includes bibliographical references (pages 161-170) and index.

Mental health disorders sourcebook: basic consumer health information about healthy brain functioning and mental illnesses including depression, bipolar disorder, anxiety disorders, posttraumatic stress disorder, obsessive-compulsive disorder, psychotic and personality disorders, eating disorders, impulse control disorders, and more; along with information about medications and treatments, mental health Concerns in specific groups such as children, adolescents, older adults, minority populations, and lesbian, gay, bisexual, and transsexual, a glossary of related terms, and directories of resources for additional help and information

LCCN	2021033373
Type of material	Book
Main title	Mental health disorders sourcebook: basic consumer health information about healthy brain functioning and mental illnesses including depression, bipolar disorder, anxiety disorders, posttraumatic stress disorder, obsessive-compulsive disorder, psychotic and personality disorders, eating disorders, impulse control disorders, and more; along with information about medications and treatments, mental health Concerns in specific groups such as children, adolescents, older adults, minority populations, and lesbian, gay, bisexual, and transsexual, a glossary of related terms, and directories of resources for additional help and information / edited by Kevin Hayes.
Edition	Eighth edition.
Published/Produced	Detroit, MI: Omnigraphics, Inc., [2021]
Description	1 online resource
ISBN	9780780819719 (ebook) (library binding)
LC classification	RC454.4
Related names	Hayes, Kevin (Editor of health information), editor.
Summary	"Provides basic consumer health information about the signs, symptoms, risk factors, and treatment of various mental illnesses, and the special mental-health concerns of children and other groups, along with tips for maintaining mental wellness. Includes

	index, glossary of related terms, and other resources"-- Provided by publisher.
LC Subjects	Mental illness.
	Psychiatry.
Notes	Includes index.
Additional formats	Print version: Mental health disorders sourcebook Eighth edition. Detroit, MI: Omnigraphics, Inc., [2021] 9780780819702 (DLC) 2021033372
Series	Health reference series

Mental health disorders sourcebook: basic consumer health information about healthy brain functioning and mental illnesses including depression, bipolar disorder, anxiety disorders, posttraumatic stress disorder, obsessive-compulsive disorder, psychotic and personality disorders, eating disorders, impulse control disorders, and more; along with information about medications and treatments, mental health Concerns in specific groups such as children, adolescents, older adults, minority populations, and lesbian, gay, bisexual, and transsexual, a glossary of related terms, and directories of resources for additional help and information

LCCN	2021033372
Type of material	Book
Main title	Mental health disorders sourcebook: basic consumer health information about healthy brain functioning and mental illnesses including depression, bipolar disorder, anxiety disorders, posttraumatic stress disorder, obsessive-compulsive cisorder, psychotic and personality disorders, eating disorders, impulse control disorders, and more; along with information about medications and treatments, mental health Concerns in specific groups such as children, adolescents, older adults, minority populations, and lesbian, gay, bisexual, and transsexual, a hlossary of related terms, and directories of resources for additional help and information / edited by Kevin Hayes.
Edition	Eighth edition.
Published/Produced	Detroit, MI: Omnigraphics, Inc., [2021]

ISBN	9780780819702 (library binding) (ebook)
LC classification	RC454.4 .M458 2021
Related names	Hayes, Kevin (Editor of health information), editor.
Summary	"Provides basic consumer health information about the signs, symptoms, risk factors, and treatment of various mental illnesses, and the special mental-health concerns of children and other groups, along with tips for maintaining mental wellness. Includes index, glossary of related terms, and other resources"-- Provided by publisher.
LC Subjects	Mental illness. Psychiatry.
Notes	Includes index.
Additional formats	Online version: Mental health disorders sourcebook Eighth edition. Detroit, MI: Omnigraphics, Inc., [2021] 9780780819719 (DLC) 2021033373
Series	Health reference series

Mental health information for teens: health tips about mental wellness and mental illness: including facts about recognizing and treating mood, anxiety, personality, psychotic, behavioral, impulse control, and addiction disorders

LCCN	2021029387
Type of material	Book
Main title	Mental health information for teens: health tips about mental wellness and mental illness: including facts about recognizing and treating mood, anxiety, personality, psychotic, behavioral, impulse control, and addiction disorders / edited by Kevin Hayes.
Edition	Sixth edition.
Published/Produced	Detroit, MI: Omnigraphics, Inc., [2021]
Description	1 online resource
ISBN	9780780819269 (ebook) (library binding)
LC classification	RJ499
Related names	Hayes, Kevin (Editor of health information) editor.
Summary	"Provides consumer health information about the causes, warning signs, and symptoms of mental

	health disorders, along with facts about treatment approaches and tips for teens on coping with stress, building self-esteem, and maintaining mental wellness. Includes index and a directory of crisis helplines and related organizations"-- Provided by publisher.
LC Subjects	Teenagers--Mental health.
	Adolescent psychology.
	Child mental health.
Notes	Includes index.
Intended Audience	Ages 13 (Omnigraphics, Inc.)
	Grades 7-9 (Omnigraphics, Inc.)
Additional formats	Print version: Mental health information for teens Sixth edition. Detroit, MI: Omnigraphics, Inc., [2021] 9780780819252 (DLC) 2021029386
Series	Teen health series

Mental health information for teens: health tips about mental wellness and mental illness: including facts about recognizing and treating mood, anxiety, personality, psychotic, behavioral, impulse control, and addiction disorders

LCCN	2021029386
Type of material	Book
Main title	Mental health information for teens: health tips about mental wellness and mental illness: including facts about recognizing and treating mood, anxiety, personality, psychotic, behavioral, impulse control, and addiction disorders / edited by Kevin Hayes.
Edition	Sixth edition.
Published/Produced	Detroit, MI: Omnigraphics, Inc., [2021]
ISBN	9780780819252 (library binding)
	(ebook)
LC classification	RJ499 .M419 2021
Related names	Hayes, Kevin (Editor of health information) editor.
Summary	"Provides consumer health information about the causes, warning signs, and symptoms of mental health disorders, along with facts about treatment approaches and tips for teens on coping with stress, building self-esteem, and maintaining mental

	wellness. Includes index and a directory of crisis helplines and related organizations"-- Provided by publisher.
LC Subjects	Teenagers--Mental health.
	Adolescent psychology.
	Child mental health.
Notes	Includes index.
Intended Audience	Ages 13 (Omnigraphics, Inc.)
	Grades 7-9 (Omnigraphics, Inc.)
Additional formats	Online version: Mental health information for teens Sixth edition. Detroit, MI: Omnigraphics, [2021] 9780780819269 (DLC) 2021029387
Series	Teen health series

Mental patient: psychiatric ethics from a patient's perspective

LCCN	2021052789
Type of material	Book
Personal name	Gosselin, Abigail, 1977- author.
Main title	Mental patient: psychiatric ethics from a patient's perspective / Abigail Gosselin.
Published/Produced	Cambridge, Massachusetts: The MIT Press, [2022]
ISBN	9780262544313 (paperback)
LC classification	RC454
Summary	"A philosopher explains how it feels to undergo a psychotic break and what mental health professionals need to know to assist recovery"-- Provided by publisher.
Contents	Psychosis - Autonomy - Patient - Trust - Empathy - Testimony - Meaning-Making - Choices.
Other Subjects	Gosselin, Abigail, 1977-
	Psychotic Disorders--psychology
	Mentally Ill Persons--psychology
	Professional-Patient Relations
	Personal Autonomy
	Therapeutic Alliance
	Patient Compliance--psychology
Form/Genre	Personal Narrative
Notes	Includes bibliographical references and index.

Series	Basic bioethics
	Basic bioethics

Pathophysiology, physical assessment, and pharmacology: advanced integrative clinical concepts

LCCN	2021023454
Type of material	Book
Personal name	Best, Janie T. author.
Main title	Pathophysiology, physical assessment, and pharmacology: advanced integrative clinical concepts / Janie T. Best, Grace Buttriss, Annette Hines.
Published/Produced	Philadelphia: F.A. Davis Company, [2022]
Description	1 online resource
ISBN	9780803675742 (ebook)
	(paperback)
LC classification	RT48
Related names	Buttriss, Grace, author.
	Hines, Annette, author.
Summary	"This groundbreaking textbook, Pathophysiology, Physical Assessment, and Pharmacology: Advanced Integrative Clinical Concepts, facilitates knowledge in a way that enables student understanding for real world application. Integrating the concepts of physiology/ pathophysiology, physical assessment, and pharmacology eliminates the silo approach to nursing education and guides the student to explore how each element impacts the other"-- Provided by publisher.
Contents	Hypertension - Diabetes Mellitus - Obesity - IBS and IBD - Myocardial Infarction - Case Study 1 (Adult): Glaucoma - Hypertensive Disorders of Pregnancy - Gestational Diabetes - High-Risk Pregnancy - Gastrointestinal Conditions - Case Study 2 (Maternity): Vaginal Bleeding - Hyperbilirubinemia in the Newborn - Congenital Heart Disease - Respiratory Conditions - Prematurity and Newborn Conditions - Case Study 3 (Newborn): Nutrition - Asthma - Allergic and Hypersensitivity Disorders -

	Gastroesophageal Reflux Disease - Traumatic Brain Injury - Otitis Media - Case Study 4 (Pediatrics): Acute Lymphoblastic Leukemia - Healthy Aging - Heart Failure - Pneumonia - Osteoarthritis and Rheumatoid Arthritis - Chronic Kidney Disease - Case Study 5 (Geriatric): Osteoporosis - Altered Cognitive Function - Anxiety and Depression - Psychotic Disorders - Substance Abuse Disorders - Case Study 6 (Mental Health): ADHD.
Other Subjects	Nursing Process
	Nursing Care
Notes	Includes bibliographical references.
Additional formats	Print version: Best, Janie T. Pathophysiology, physical assessment, and pharmacology Philadelphia: F.A. Davis Company, [2022] 9780803675674 (DLC) 2021023453

Pathophysiology, physical assessment, and pharmacology: advanced integrative clinical concepts

LCCN	2021023453
Type of material	Book
Personal name	Best, Janie T. author.
Main title	Pathophysiology, physical assessment, and pharmacology: advanced integrative clinical concepts / Janie T. Best, Grace Buttriss, Annette Hines.
Published/Produced	Philadelphia: F.A. Davis Company, [2022]
ISBN	9780803675674 (paperback)
	(ebook)
LC classification	RT48
Related names	Buttriss, Grace, author.
	Hines, Annette, author.
Summary	"This groundbreaking textbook, Pathophysiology, Physical Assessment, and Pharmacology: Advanced Integrative Clinical Concepts, facilitates knowledge in a way that enables student understanding for real world application. Integrating the concepts of physiology/ pathophysiology, physical assessment, and pharmacology eliminates the silo approach to

Contents	nursing education and guides the student to explore how each element impacts the other"-- Provided by publisher. Hypertension - Diabetes Mellitus - Obesity - IBS and IBD - Myocardial Infarction - Case Study 1 (Adult): Glaucoma - Hypertensive Disorders of Pregnancy - Gestational Diabetes - High-Risk Pregnancy - Gastrointestinal Conditions - Case Study 2 (Maternity): Vaginal Bleeding - Hyperbilirubinemia in the Newborn - Congenital Heart Disease - Respiratory Conditions - Prematurity and Newborn Conditions - Case Study 3 (Newborn): Nutrition - Asthma - Allergic and Hypersensitivity Disorders - Gastroesophageal Reflux Disease - Traumatic Brain Injury - Otitis Media - Case Study 4 (Pediatrics): Acute Lymphoblastic Leukemia - Healthy Aging - Heart Failure - Pneumonia - Osteoarthritis and Rheumatoid Arthritis - Chronic Kidney Disease - Case Study 5 (Geriatric): Osteoporosis - Altered Cognitive Function - Anxiety and Depression - Psychotic Disorders - Substance Abuse Disorders - Case Study 6 (Mental Health): ADHD.
Other Subjects	Nursing Process Nursing Care
Notes	Includes bibliographical references.
Additional formats	Online version: Best, Janie T. Pathophysiology, physical assessment, and pharmacology First. Philadelphia: F.A. Davis Company, [2022] 9780803675742 (DLC) 2021023454

Postpartum mental health disorders: a casebook

LCCN	2019053081
Type of material	Book
Main title	Postpartum mental health disorders: a casebook / editors, Gail Erlick Robinson, Carol C. Nadelson, Gisele Apter.
Published/Produced	New York, NY: Oxford University Press, [2020]
Description	1 online resource
ISBN	9780190929619 (ebook)

Bibliography

	9780190849979 (epub)
	(paperback)
LC classification	RG852
Related names	Robinson, Gail Erlick, editor.
	Nadelson, Carol C., editor.
	Apter, Gisele, editor.
Summary	"Postpartum Mental Health Disorders: A Casebook describes the recognition and management of psychiatric disorders that present in the postpartum period. Case vignettes illustrate the type of complaints that may present to the psychiatrist, primary care physician, obstetrician, nurse practitioner, doula or other health care professionals. Chapters cover depression, anxiety disorders, obsessive compulsive disorder (OCD), psychotic disorders, bipolar disorders, posttraumatic stress disorders, personality disorders and drug abuse. Each chapter includes information about differential and provisional diagnoses, epidemiology, treatment and prognosis with advice as to when to refer to a specialist. More general chapters address risk factors for developing postpartum disorders, prevention and the uses and safety of psychotropic medication during breastfeeding. Two frequently used screening questionnaires are included with instructions as to use. Some key references or links are included"-- Provided by publisher.
Contents	Risks for a Postpartum Disorder - Postpartum Adaptation: Normal; Baby Blues; Baby Pinks - Postpartum Depression - Postpartum Anxiety - Postpartum Psychosis - Postpartum Obsessive-Compulsive Disorder - Traumatic Childbirth and Postpartum Posttraumatic Stress Disorder - Personality Disorders in the Postpartum - Disorders of Attachment - Eating Disorders in the Postpartum Period - Prevention of Postpartum Disorders - Psychopharmacology in Pregnancy and Breastfeeding.
Other Subjects	Mental Disorders

	Postpartum Period
	Pregnancy Complications
Form/Genre	Case Reports
Notes	Includes bibliographical references and index.
Additional formats	Print version: Postpartum mental health disorders New York, NY: Oxford University Press, [2020] 9780190849955 (DLC) 2019053080

Postpartum mental health disorders: a casebook

LCCN	2019053080
Type of material	Book
Main title	Postpartum mental health disorders: a casebook / editors, Gail Erlick Robinson, Carol C. Nadelson, Gisele Apter.
Published/Produced	New York, NY: Oxford University Press, [2020]
ISBN	9780190849955 (paperback)
	(epub)
	(ebook)
LC classification	RG852
Related names	Robinson, Gail Erlick, editor.
	Nadelson, Carol C., editor.
	Apter, Gisele, editor.
Summary	"Postpartum Mental Health Disorders: A Casebook describes the recognition and management of psychiatric disorders that present in the postpartum period. Case vignettes illustrate the type of complaints that may present to the psychiatrist, primary care physician, obstetrician, nurse practitioner, doula or other health care professionals. Chapters cover depression, anxiety disorders, obsessive compulsive disorder (OCD), psychotic disorders, bipolar disorders, posttraumatic stress disorders, personality disorders and drug abuse. Each chapter includes information about differential and provisional diagnoses, epidemiology, treatment and prognosis with advice as to when to refer to a specialist. More general chapters address risk factors for developing postpartum disorders, prevention and the uses and safety of psychotropic medication during

	breastfeeding. Two frequently used screening questionnaires are included with instructions as to use. Some key references or links are included"-- Provided by publisher.
Contents	Risks for a Postpartum Disorder - Postpartum Adaptation: Normal; Baby Blues; Baby Pinks - Postpartum Depression - Postpartum Anxiety - Postpartum Psychosis - Postpartum Obsessive-Compulsive Disorder - Traumatic Childbirth and Postpartum Posttraumatic Stress Disorder - Personality Disorders in the Postpartum - Disorders of Attachment - Eating Disorders in the Postpartum Period - Prevention of Postpartum Disorders - Psychopharmacology in Pregnancy and Breastfeeding.
Other Subjects	Mental Disorders
	Postpartum Period
	Pregnancy Complications
Form/Genre	Case Reports
Notes	Includes bibliographical references and index.
Additional formats	Online version: Postpartum mental health disorders. New York, NY: Oxford University Press, [2020] 9780190849979 (DLC) 2019053081

Prescribing together: a relational guide to psychopharmacology

LCCN	2021010593
Type of material	Book
Personal name	Kinghorn, Warren A., author.
Main title	Prescribing together: a relational guide to psychopharmacology / Warren A. Kinghorn, Abraham M. Nussbaum.
Edition	First edition.
Published/Produced	Washington, DC: American Psychiatric Association Publishing, [2021]
Description	1 online resource
ISBN	9781615372898 (ebook)
	(paperback; alk. paper)
LC classification	RC483.3
Related names	Nussbaum, Abraham M., 1975- author.

American Psychiatric Association Publishing, publisher.

Summary

"What if, rather than being dispensers of medication, mental health clinicians and primary care providers treating mental disorders were collaborators with patients in the prescribing relationship? To prescribe more effectively and achieve health equity, Warren Kinghorn and Abraham Nussbaum argue, it's necessary-and in Prescribing Together, they offer a roadmap for making it a reality. In these pages, readers will find practical introductions to key concepts, from cultural formation and structural competency to collaborative deprescribing, and profiles, enlivened by personal anecdotes, of a diverse group of accomplished clinicians that offer evidence-based strategies for building strong alliances in the context of 13 mental disorder categories, including generalized anxiety disorder, major depressive disorder, borderline personality disorder, and neurocognitive disorders. By focusing on how, rather than what, to prescribe, this book makes room for patients' lived experiences and interpersonal and social contexts, returning to them a sense of agency and empowering them to set meaningful goals and be active participants in their own flourishing"-- Provided by publisher.

Contents

Introduction: From Dispensers to Collaborators - Relationship Matters - Prescribing Alliances - Peak Performance: Prescribing in the Context of Attention-Deficit/Hyperactivity Disorder - Visions and Voices: Prescribing in the Context of Schizophrenia and Other Psychotic Disorders - Stabilization Forces: Prescribing in the Context of Bipolar Disorder - Frayed Edges: Prescribing in the Context of Depressive and Anxiety Disorders - Unwelcome Strangers: Prescribing in the Context of Obsessive-Compulsive and Related Disorders - Building Peace: Prescribing in the Context of Trauma- and Stressor-Related Disorders - When the Body Speaks:

	Prescribing in the Context of Somatic Distress - Befriending the Body: Prescribing in the Context of Eating Disorders - Getting Clean: Prescribing in the Context of Substance Use Disorders - Knowing and Being Known: Prescribing in the Context of Neurocognitive Disorders - Strong Emotions: Prescribing in the Context of Borderline Personality Disorder.
Other Subjects	Mental Disorders--drug therapy
	Therapeutic Alliance
	Drug Prescriptions
	Psychotropic Drugs
Notes	Includes bibliographical references and index.
Additional formats	Print version: Kinghorn, Warren A.. Prescribing together First edition. Washington, DC: American Psychiatric Association Publishing, [2021] 9781615372881 (DLC) 2021010592

Prescribing together: a relational guide to psychopharmacology

LCCN	2021010592
Type of material	Book
Personal name	Kinghorn, Warren A., author.
Main title	Prescribing together: a relational guide to psychopharmacology / Warren A. Kinghorn, Abraham M. Nussbaum.
Edition	First edition.
Published/Produced	Washington, DC: American Psychiatric Association Publishing, [2021]
Description	x, 285 pages: illustrations; 21 cm
ISBN	9781615372881 (paperback; alk. paper)
	(ebook)
LC classification	RC483.3 .K56 2021
Related names	Nussbaum, Abraham M., 1975- author.
	American Psychiatric Association Publishing, publisher.
Summary	"What if, rather than being dispensers of medication, mental health clinicians and primary care providers treating mental disorders were collaborators with patients in the prescribing relationship? To prescribe

more effectively and achieve health equity, Warren Kinghorn and Abraham Nussbaum argue, it's necessary-and in Prescribing Together, they offer a roadmap for making it a reality. In these pages, readers will find practical introductions to key concepts, from cultural formation and structural competency to collaborative deprescribing, and profiles, enlivened by personal anecdotes, of a diverse group of accomplished clinicians that offer evidence-based strategies for building strong alliances in the context of 13 mental disorder categories, including generalized anxiety disorder, major depressive disorder, borderline personality disorder, and neurocognitive disorders. By focusing on how, rather than what, to prescribe, this book makes room for patients' lived experiences and interpersonal and social contexts, returning to them a sense of agency and empowering them to set meaningful goals and be active participants in their own flourishing"-- Provided by publisher.

Contents

Introduction: From Dispensers to Collaborators - Relationship Matters - Prescribing Alliances - Peak Performance: Prescribing in the Context of Attention-Deficit/Hyperactivity Disorder - Visions and Voices: Prescribing in the Context of Schizophrenia and Other Psychotic Disorders - Stabilization Forces: Prescribing in the Context of Bipolar Disorder - Frayed Edges: Prescribing in the Context of Depressive and Anxiety Disorders - Unwelcome Strangers: Prescribing in the Context of Obsessive-Compulsive and Related Disorders - Building Peace: Prescribing in the Context of Trauma- and Stressor-Related Disorders - When the Body Speaks: Prescribing in the Context of Somatic Distress - Befriending the Body: Prescribing in the Context of Eating Disorders - Getting Clean: Prescribing in the Context of Substance Use Disorders - Knowing and Being Known: Prescribing in the Context of Neurocognitive Disorders - Strong Emotions:

	Prescribing in the Context of Borderline Personality Disorder.
Other Subjects	Mental Disorders--drug therapy
	Therapeutic Alliance
	Drug Prescriptions
	Psychotropic Drugs
Notes	Includes bibliographical references and index.
Additional formats	Online version: Kinghorn, Warren A., Prescribing together First edition. Washington, DC: American Psychiatric Association Publishing, [2021] 9781615372898 (DLC) 2021010593

Psychiatric and mental health nursing in the UK

LCCN	2021303240
Type of material	Book
Main title	Psychiatric and mental health nursing in the UK / edited by Katie Evans, RN, BA, MLitSt, PhD, Mental Health Education Consultant, Debra Nizette, RN, DipAppSc (Nursing Ed), BAppSc (Nursing), MNursSt, Credentialed MHN, FACN, FACMHN, Director of Nursing, Queensland Health, Queensland, Australia, Anthony O'Brien, RN, BA, MPhil (Hons), PhD, FNZMHN, Senior Lecturer in Mental Health Nursing, University of Auckland; Nurse Specialist in Liaison Psychiatry, Auckland District Health Board, Auckland, New Zealand; UK adapting author, Catherine Johnson, RMN, RGN, Registered General Nurse at Guy's and St. Thomas' NHS Foundation Trust; Clinical Nurse Specialist at West London Mental Health NHS Trust, London, UK; foreword by Gemma Stacey, MN PGCHE RN (Mental Health), Associate Professor in the School of Health Sciences and Program Lead for Graduate Entry Nursing, University of Nottingham; Lecturer in Mental Health and Social Care, School of Nursing, Midwifery and Physiotherapy, University of Nottingham, Derby Education Centre, London Road Community Hospital, Derby, UK.
Published/Produced	Edinburgh: Elsevier, 2020.

Description	xiii, 546 pages: illustrations; 28 cm
ISBN	9780702080241 (paperback)
	0702080241
LC classification	RC440 .P7294 2020
Related names	Evans, Katie (Psychiatric nurse), editor.
	Nizette, Debra, editor.
	O'Brien, Anthony J., editor.
	Johnson, Catherine, RGN, editor.
Summary	'Psychiatric and Mental Health Nursing in the UK' is an adaptation of Australia and New Zealand's foremost mental health nursing text and is an essential resource for both mental health nursing students and qualified nurses. It has been thoroughly revised and updated to reflect current research and the UK guidelines, as well as the changing attitudes about mental health, mental health services and mental health nursing in UK. Set within a recovery and patient framework, the text provides vital information for approaching the most familiar disorders mental health nurses and students will see in clinical practice, along with helpful suggestions about what the mental health nurse can say and do to interact effectively with patients and their families
Incomplete contents	PART 1 Preparing for psychiatric and mental health nursing The effective nurse Recovery as the context for practice Historical foundations Professional, legal and ethical issues Settings for mental health PART 2 Influences on mental health Mental health theory and influence across the lifespan Trauma, crisis, loss and grief Physical health PART 3 The people with whom mental health nurses work Mental health and wellness Working with families in mental health Disorders of childhood and adolescence Mental disorders of older age Learning disabilities Forensic mental health nursing PART 4 Mental disorders that people experience Schizophrenia and psychotic disorders Mood disorders Personality disorders Anxiety, trauma and stress-related disorders Eating disorders Substance use and comorbid mental health

	disorders PART 5 What mental health nurses can do to help Mental health promotion, prevention and primary healthcare Assessment in mental health nursing Challenging behaviour, risk and responses Therapeutic interventions Psychopharmacology Glossary Index
LC Subjects	Psychiatric nursing--Great Britain.
Other Subjects	Psychiatric Nursing.
	Health and Fitness.
	Psychiatric nursing.
	Health and Wellbeing.
	United Kingdom.
	Great Britain.
Notes	Includes bibliographical references and index.

Psychiatry: pretest self-assessment and review

LCCN	2020029794
Type of material	Book
Personal name	Klamen, Debra L., author.
Main title	Psychiatry: pretest self-assessment and review / Debra L. Klamen.
Edition	15th edition.
Published/Produced	New York: McGraw Hill, [2021]
ISBN	9781260467413 (paperback)
	(ebook)
LC classification	RC480.5
Summary	"PreTest: Psychiatry is part of the successful PreTest clinical series, offering hundreds of Board style questions designed to help you in your clerkship and on the shelf exam. Completely revised to reflect new trends, findings and practices, all questions reflect both the format and range of content you'll be responsible for knowing during your clerkship and on your shelf exam. Each question is accompanied by a detailed answer that highlights important information and explains why each answer choice is right or wrong. To ensure that all content, was relevant, timely and high yield, this edition was carefully reviewed and edited by medical students who have

Contents	successfully mastered their clerkship"-- Provided by publisher. Basics of Psychiatry - Biologic and Related Sciences - Disorders Seen in Childhood and Adolescence - Neurocognitive Disorders and Consultation-Liaison Psychiatry - Schizophrenia and Other Psychotic Disorders - Mood Disorders - Anxiety Disorders, Obsessive-Compulsive, Trauma- or Stress-Related Disorders - Somatic Symptom and Dissociative Disorders - Personality Disorders - Human Sexuality, Sleep and Other Disorders - Substance-Related Disorders - Management of Psychiatric Disorders - Law and Ethics in Psychiatry - Self-Test, Uncued Study Questions.
Other Subjects	Mental Disorders
	Psychotherapy
Form/Genre	Examination Questions
Notes	Includes bibliographical references and index.

Psychoanalysis in medicine: applying psychoanalytic thought to contemporary medical care

LCCN	2020018878
Type of material	Book
Personal name	Steinberg, Paul Ian, author.
Main title	Psychoanalysis in medicine: applying psychoanalytic thought to contemporary medical care / Paul Ian Steinberg.
Published/Produced	New York, NY: Routledge Taylor & Francis Group, 2021.
Description	1 online resource.
ISBN	9780429031885 (ebook)
	(hardback)
	(paperback)
LC classification	RC454.4
Summary	"This book shows how contemporary psychoanalytic thinking can be applied in the everyday practice of medicine to enhance the practice of family medicine and all clinical specialties. Dr. Steinberg analyzes his writings over the past 35 years-on psychiatry and

family medicine, liaison psychiatry, and supervision and mentoring-based on developments in psychoanalytic thinking. Divided into sections based on different venues of medical practice, including family medicine clinics, inpatient medical and surgical units, and psychiatric inpatient units and outpatient programs, chapters illustrate how various concepts in psychoanalysis can enhance physicians' understanding and management of their patients. A concluding section contains applications of psychoanalytic thought in nonclinical areas pertinent to medicine, including preventing suicide among physicians, residents and medical students, sexual abuse of patients by physicians, and oral examination anxiety in physicians. Readers will learn to apply psychoanalytic concepts with a rational approach that enhances their understanding and management of their patients and practice of medicine generally"-- Provided by publisher.

Contents

"Problem Patients": Patients with Significant Personality Disturbance - Interviewing the Patient - "Are All My Patients Depressed?": The (Mis-)diagnosis of Depression - "My Patient is Psychotic": Dealing with a Patient with a Paranoid Delusion about Her Disease - Holding Patients with Medication: Using Neuroleptics as an Adjunct to Psychotherapy in the Patients with Severe Personality Disorders - What Psychoanalysis and Psychiatry Offer to Medicine - Psychoanalytic Approaches to Psychosomatic Medicine - Psychiatry for the Masses: Broader Indications for Psychiatric Consultation - Where Does My Patient Fit In? Organizing One's Diagnostic Thinking In Differentiating Patients according to their Symptoms - "The Most Unkindest Cut of All": Psychiatric Complications of Surgery in Men - Psychiatric Diagnosis is not a Diagnosis of Exclusion: A Patient with Insulinoma Presenting for Psychiatric Assessment - Differentiating Psychiatric and Medical Conditions: A Case of Hyperthyroidism

Bibliography

	Presenting as Delusional Disorder - "My Patient is Hysterical": Adrenal Carcinoma and Hypertension Presenting with Catatonic Stupor - The Mother Who Couldn't Name Her Child: Problems of Attachment, Identity and The Capacity to Think - Freud on the Ward: Integration of Psychoanalytic Concepts in the Formulation and Management of Hospitalized Psychiatric Patients - Psychoanalytic Approaches Integrated into Day Treatment and Inpatient Settings - Attack of Nerves: Oral Examination Anxiety in Physicians - Healers Caring for Themselves and Each Other: Preventing Suicide in Medical Students, Residents and Ourselves - Professional Betrayal: Sexual Abuse of Adult Female Patients by Male Physicians.
Other Subjects	Psychoanalytic Theory Psychoanalytic Therapy Primary Health Care Mental Disorders--diagnosis Mental Disorders--therapy Psychology, Medical
Notes	Includes bibliographical references and index.
Additional formats	Print version: Steinberg, Paul Ian. Psychoanalysis in medicine New York, NY: Routledge Taylor & Francis Group, 2021. 9780367144050 (DLC) 2020018877

Psychoanalysis in medicine: applying psychoanalytic thought to contemporary medical care

LCCN	2020018877
Type of material	Book
Personal name	Steinberg, Paul Ian, author.
Main title	Psychoanalysis in medicine: applying psychoanalytic thought to contemporary medical care / Paul Ian Steinberg.
Published/Produced	New York: Routledge, 2021.
Description	xi, 229 pages; 23 cm
ISBN	9780367144050 (hardback) 9780367144067 (paperback)

LC classification	(ebook) RC454.4 .S725 2021
Summary	"This book shows how contemporary psychoanalytic thinking can be applied in the everyday practice of medicine to enhance the practice of family medicine and all clinical specialties. Dr. Steinberg analyzes his writings over the past 35 years-on psychiatry and family medicine, liaison psychiatry, and supervision and mentoring-based on developments in psychoanalytic thinking. Divided into sections based on different venues of medical practice, including family medicine clinics, inpatient medical and surgical units, and psychiatric inpatient units and outpatient programs, chapters illustrate how various concepts in psychoanalysis can enhance physicians' understanding and management of their patients. A concluding section contains applications of psychoanalytic thought in nonclinical areas pertinent to medicine, including preventing suicide among physicians, residents and medical students, sexual abuse of patients by physicians, and oral examination anxiety in physicians. Readers will learn to apply psychoanalytic concepts with a rational approach that enhances their understanding and management of their patients and practice of medicine generally"-- Provided by publisher.
Contents	"Problem Patients": Patients with Significant Personality Disturbance - Interviewing the Patient - "Are All My Patients Depressed?": The (Mis-)diagnosis of Depression - "My Patient is Psychotic": Dealing with a Patient with a Paranoid Delusion about Her Disease - Holding Patients with Medication: Using Neuroleptics as an Adjunct to Psychotherapy in the Patients with Severe Personality Disorders - What Psychoanalysis and Psychiatry Offer to Medicine - Psychoanalytic Approaches to Psychosomatic Medicine - Psychiatry for the Masses: Broader Indications for Psychiatric Consultation - Where Does My Patient Fit In? Organizing One's

	Diagnostic Thinking In Differentiating Patients according to their Symptoms - "The Most Unkindest Cut of All": Psychiatric Complications of Surgery in Men - Psychiatric Diagnosis is not a Diagnosis of Exclusion: A Patient with Insulinoma Presenting for Psychiatric Assessment - Differentiating Psychiatric and Medical Conditions: A Case of Hyperthyroidism Presenting as Delusional Disorder - "My Patient is Hysterical": Adrenal Carcinoma and Hypertension Presenting with Catatonic Stupor - The Mother Who Couldn't Name Her Child: Problems of Attachment, Identity and The Capacity to Think - Freud on the Ward: Integration of Psychoanalytic Concepts in the Formulation and Management of Hospitalized Psychiatric Patients - Psychoanalytic Approaches Integrated into Day Treatment and Inpatient Settings - Attack of Nerves: Oral Examination Anxiety in Physicians - Healers Caring for Themselves and Each Other: Preventing Suicide in Medical Students, Residents and Ourselves - Professional Betrayal: Sexual Abuse of Adult Female Patients by Male Physicians.
Other Subjects	Psychoanalytic Theory
	Psychoanalytic Therapy
	Primary Health Care
	Mental Disorders--diagnosis
	Mental Disorders--therapy
	Psychology, Medical
Notes	Includes bibliographical references and index.
Additional formats	Online version: Steinberg, Paul Ian, Psychoanalysis in medicine New York, NY: Routledge, 2021. 9780429031885 (DLC) 2020018878

Psychopharmacology: straight talk on mental health medications

LCCN	2021005456
Type of material	Book
Personal name	Wegmann, Joseph, author.
Main title	Psychopharmacology: straight talk on mental health medications / Joe Wegmann.

Edition	Fourth edition.
Published/Produced	Eau Claire, WI: PESI Publishing, [2021]
ISBN	9781683732983 (paperback)
	(ebk)
LC classification	RM315
Summary	"This is the definitive guide and desk reference for healthcare professionals and patients to expand their knowledge in the pharmacological and behavioral treatment of psychosis, anxiety, depression, bipolar, insomnia and ADHD"-- Provided by publisher.
Contents	The DSM®; Medical Model; Neurobiology - The First Visits with the Client - Schizophrenia and Other Psychotic Spectrum Disorders - Depression - Bipolar Disorder - The Many Manifestations of Anxiety - Opiates, Opioids and Medical Marijuana - Antipsychotics - Antidepressants - Treatment-Resistant Depression - Other Treatment Paths for Managing Depression - Mood-Stabilizing Agents - Dosage Range Chart-Mood Stabilizers - Anticonvulsants - Antianxiety Medications, Sleep Agents - Dosage Range Chart-Antianxiety Medications, - Sleep Agents - Anxiety and Insomnia: Treatment Beyond Medication - Treatment of Opiate and Opioid Disorders - Chronic Pain Management - Specific Population Groups - Attention Deficit Hyperactivity Disorder - Herbals and Supplements - Solving Medication Challenges - Psychopharmacology Going Forward.
Other Subjects	Mental Disorders--drug therapy
	Psychotropic Drugs--therapeutic use
	Psychotherapy
Notes	Includes bibliographical references and index.

Psychopharmacology algorithms: clinical guidance from the Psychopharmacology Algorithm Project at the Harvard South Shore Psychiatry Residency Program

LCCN	2020018487
Type of material	Book

Main title	Psychopharmacology algorithms: clinical guidance from the Psychopharmacology Algorithm Project at the Harvard South Shore Psychiatry Residency Program / [edited by] David N. Osser.
Published/Produced	Philadelphia: Wolters Kluwer Health, [2021]
ISBN	9781975151195 (paperback)
LC classification	RC483
Related names	Osser, David N. (David Neal), editor.
Summary	"Algorithms are useful in the field of psychopharmacology as they can serve as guidelines for avoiding the biases and cognitive lapses that are common when treating conditions that rely on uncertain data. In spite of this, evidence-based practices in psychopharmacology often require years to become widely adopted. The Psychopharmacology Algorithm Project at Harvard's South Shore Medical Program is an effort to speed up the adoption of evidence-based research into the day-to-day treatment of patients"-- Provided by publisher.
Contents	On the Value of Evidence-Based Psychopharmacology Algorithms / David N. Osser, Robert D. Patterson - The Psychopharmacology Algorithm Project at the Harvard South Shore Program: An Update on Unipolar Nonpsychotic Depression / Christoforos Iraklis Giakoumatos and David Osser - The Psychopharmacology Algorithm Project at the Harvard South Shore Program: An Update on Bipolar Depression / Arash Ansari and David N. Osser - The Psychopharmacology Algorithm Project at the Harvard South Shore Program: An Algorithm for Acute Mania / Othman Mohammad and David N. Osser - The Psychopharmacology Algorithm Project at the Harvard South Shore Program: Update on Psychotic Depression / Michael Tang, David N. Osser - The Psychopharmacology Algorithm Project at the Harvard South Shore Program: An Update on Schizophrenia / David N. Osser, Mohsen Jalali Roudsari, and Theo Manschreck - The Psychopharmacology Algorithm Project at the

	Harvard South Shore Program: An Algorithm for Generalized Anxiety Disorder / Harmony Raylen Abejuel, and David N. Osser - The Psychopharmacology Algorithm Project at The Harvard South Shore Program: An Update on Generalized Social Anxiety Disorder / David N. Osser and Lance R. Dunlop - The Psychopharmacology Algorithm Project at the Harvard South Shore Program: An Update on Posttraumatic Stress Disorder / Laura A. Bajor, Ana Nectara Ticlea, and David N. Osser - The Psychopharmacology Algorithm Project at the Harvard South Shore Program: An algorithm for adults with obsessive-compulsive disorder / Ashley M. Beaulieua, Edward Tabaskyb, David N. Osser - Pharmacologic Approach to the Psychiatric Inpatient / Arash Ansari, David N. Osser, Leonard S. Lai, Paul M. Schoenfeld, and Kenneth C. Potts - Guidelines, Algorithms, and Evidence-Based Psychopharmacology Training for Psychiatric Residents / David N. Osser, Robert D. Patterson, James J. Levitt.
Other Subjects	Psychopharmacology Algorithm Project at the Harvard South Shore Psychiatry Residency Program. Mental Disorders--drug therapy Psychotropic Drugs--administration & dosage Algorithms Practice Guidelines as Topic Evidence-Based Medicine
Notes	Includes bibliographical references and index.

Psychotic disorders: comprehensive conceptualization and treatments

LCCN	2019055817
Type of material	Book
Main title	Psychotic disorders: comprehensive conceptualization and treatments / editors, Carol A Tamminga, Elena I. Ivleva, Ulrich Reininghaus, Jim van Os.
Published/Produced	New York, NY: Oxford University Press, [2021]
Description	1 online resource

ISBN	9780190653293 (epub)
	9780197501467 (ebook)
	(hardback)
LC classification	RC55
Related names	Tamminga, Carol A, editor.
	Ivleva, Elena I., editor.
	Reininghaus, Ulrich, editor.
	Os, J. van (Jim van), editor.
Summary	"The definition of psychotic spectrum disorders such as schizophrenia has evolved with changing nosogy and scientific advancements over the last 200 years. Understanding both the historical evolution of the concept as well as recent changes reflected in the American Psychiatric Association's Diagnostic and Statistical Manual (DSM-5) as well as the National Institute of Health's (NIH) Research Domain Criteria (RDOC) framework are critical for informing current efforts to further update and refine the nosology of psychotic spectrum disorders. This chapter offers an overview of past classification schemes, current standards, and novel approaches to further improve the validity of these definitions through use of biomarkers, reverse nosologies, and digital phenotyping tools like smartphones and sensors"-- Provided by publisher.
Other Subjects	Psychotic Disorders
	Psychotic Disorders--therapy
Notes	Includes bibliographical references and index.
Additional formats	Print version: Psychotic disorders New York, NY: Oxford University Press, [2021] 9780190653279 (DLC) 2019055816

Psychotic disorders: comprehensive conceptualization and treatments

LCCN	2019055816
Type of material	Book
Main title	Psychotic disorders: comprehensive conceptualization and treatments / editors, Carol A Tamminga, Elena I. Ivleva, Ulrich Reininghaus, Jim van Os.

Published/Produced	New York, NY: Oxford University Press, [2021]
ISBN	9780190653279 (hardback)
	(epub)
	(ebook)
LC classification	RC55
Related names	Tamminga, Carol A, editor.
	Ivleva, Elena I., editor.
	Reininghaus, Ulrich, editor.
	Os, J. van (Jim van), editor.
Summary	"The definition of psychotic spectrum disorders such as schizophrenia has evolved with changing nosogy and scientific advancements over the last 200 years. Understanding both the historical evolution of the concept as well as recent changes reflected in the American Psychiatric Association's Diagnostic and Statistical Manual (DSM-5) as well as the National Institute of Health's (NIH) Research Domain Criteria (RDOC) framework are critical for informing current efforts to further update and refine the nosology of psychotic spectrum disorders. This chapter offers an overview of past classification schemes, current standards, and novel approaches to further improve the validity of these definitions through use of biomarkers, reverse nosologies, and digital phenotyping tools like smartphones and sensors"-- Provided by publisher.
Other Subjects	Psychotic Disorders
	Psychotic Disorders--therapy
Notes	Includes bibliographical references and index.
Additional formats	Online version: Psychotic disorders New York, NY: Oxford University Press, [2021] 9780190653293 (DLC) 2019055817

Salvation and the soundness of mind

LCCN	2021938084
Type of material	Book
Personal name	Whitehead, Miriam, author.
Main title	Salvation and the soundness of mind / Miriam Whitehead.

Published/Produced	Lanham: Broad Wing Press, 2021.
ISBN	9781938373534 (paperback)
	(ebook)
Summary	"God's grace and mercy has been exceedingly abundant in my life. I have been diagnosed as Bipolar, with psychotic disorders. I have attempted suicide and I also have a history of Obsessive-Compulsive Disorder, and anxiety attacks. I have been prescribed medication to alter my behavior and mood. Some of the medication was helpful but some was not. I have learned that when I'm in the will of God, my mind is stable. When I go on my own path and step out of the Lord's plan, I have issues. The Lord has provided men and women with gifts and talents to help people like myself and others. I appreciate people who have the gift of hearing and listening. These men and women are resources for a sound mind. Just as the Lord provides rain as a resource for flowers and trees. It is my prayer that this book would provide scriptures, testimonials, and prophetic words to help combat the woes of the mind and to incite change and freedom. "Before you can be free you have to acknowledge you are bound"--Provided by publisher.

Strengthening the DSM: incorporating intersectionality, resilience, and cultural competence

LCCN	2020041721
Type of material	Book
Personal name	Garcia, Betty, 1943- author.
Main title	Strengthening the DSM: incorporating intersectionality, resilience, and cultural competence / Betty Garcia, Randy Nedegaard, John-Paul "JP" Legerski.
Edition	Third edition.
Published/Produced	New York: Springer Publishing Company, [2021]
Description	1 online resource
ISBN	9780826164360 (Instructor's PowerPoints) (paperback)

	(Instructor's Manual)
	9780826164452 (ebook)
	(Instructor's Syllabus)
LC classification	RC469
Related names	Nedegaard, Randy, author.
	Legerski, John-Paul, author.
Summary	"A major challenge with the utilization of the DSM is to introduce diagnostic protocols that support systematic inquiry on significant diagnostic information that was gathered via the multiaxial system that was first introduced in the DSM-III, used for 33 years, and was eventually removed in the DSM-5. An additional challenge is for the clinician is to find assessment formulations that address the whole person in his or her real-life contexts related to a vast variety of aspects of their social identity such as gender identity, culture, ethnicity/race, and socioeconomic class. These diverse sources of strength and resiliency to counterbalance sources of stress are essential in a person first approach to clinical practice."-- Provided by publisher.
Contents	A Conceptual Framework for the Intersectionality/ Resiliency Formulation - Adding Intersectionality and Resiliency to the Diagnostic Process: A Formulation - Depressive and Bipolar Disorders - Anxiety Disorders - Traumatic and Stressor-Related Disorders - Common Disorders of Childhood - Neurocognitive Disorders: Alzheimer's Disease and Traumatic Brain Injury - Schizophrenia Spectrum and Other Psychotic Disorders - Co-occurring Disorders - Emerging Perspectives for Effective Mental Health Practice in a Cultural Wars Context - Future Directions.
Other Subjects	Mental Disorders--diagnosis
	Psychiatric Status Rating Scales
	Social Identification
	Cultural Competency
	Cultural Diversity
Notes	Includes bibliographical references and index.

Additional formats	Print version: Garcia, Betty, 1943- Strengthening the DSM Third edition. New York: Springer Publishing Company, [2021] 9780826164445 (DLC) 2020041720

Strengthening the DSM: incorporating intersectionality, resilience, and cultural competence

LCCN	2020041720
Type of material	Book
Personal name	Garcia, Betty, 1943- author.
Main title	Strengthening the DSM: incorporating intersectionality, resilience, and cultural competence / Betty Garcia, PhD, LCSW, Randy Nedegaard, PhD, LCSW, LP, John-Paul Legerski, PhD, LP.
Edition	Third edition.
Published/Produced	New York: Springer Publishing, [2021]
Description	xv, 328 pages; 26 cm
ISBN	9780826164445 (paperback)
	9780826164469 (Instructor's Manual)
	9780826164366 (Instructor's Syllabus)
	(ebook)
	(Instructor's PowerPoints)
LC classification	RC451.4.A5 G37 2021
Related names	Nedegaard, Randy, author.
	Legerski, John-Paul, author.
Summary	"A major challenge with the utilization of the DSM is to introduce diagnostic protocols that support systematic inquiry on significant diagnostic information that was gathered via the multiaxial system that was first introduced in the DSM-III, used for 33 years, and was eventually removed in the DSM-5. An additional challenge is for the clinician is to find assessment formulations that address the whole person in his or her real-life contexts related to a vast variety of aspects of their social identity such as gender identity, culture, ethnicity/race, and socioeconomic class. These diverse sources of strength and resiliency to counterbalance sources of

Contents	stress are essential in a person first approach to clinical practice."-- Provided by publisher. A Conceptual Framework for the Intersectionality/Resiliency Formulation - Adding Intersectionality and Resiliency to the Diagnostic Process: A Formulation - Depressive and Bipolar Disorders - Anxiety Disorders - Traumatic and Stressor-Related Disorders - Common Disorders of Childhood - Neurocognitive Disorders: Alzheimer's Disease and Traumatic Brain Injury - Schizophrenia Spectrum and Other Psychotic Disorders - Co-occurring Disorders - Emerging Perspectives for Effective Mental Health Practice in a Cultural Wars Context - Future Directions.
Other Subjects	Mental Disorders--diagnosis Psychiatric Status Rating Scales Social Identification Cultural Competency Cultural Diversity
Notes	Includes bibliographical references and index.
Additional formats	Online version: Garcia, Betty, 1943- Strengthening the DSM Third edition. New York: Springer Publishing Company, [2021] 9780826164452 (DLC) 2020041721

Student mental health: a guide for teachers, school and district leaders, school psychologists and nurses, social workers, counselors, and parents

LCCN	2019006080
Type of material	Book
Personal name	Dikel, William, author.
Uniform title	Teacher's guide to student mental health
Main title	Student mental health: a guide for teachers, school and district leaders, school psychologists and nurses, social workers, counselors, and parents / William Dikel.
Edition	Updated and expanded.
Published/Produced	New York: W.W. Norton & Company, 2020.
Description	xvii, 366 pages; 23 cm
ISBN	9780393714128 (pbk.)

LC classification	LB3430 .D53 2020
Contents	Introduction - The clinical-behavioral spectrum - The scope of mental health disorders affecting children and adolescents - A general introduction to children's mental health - Mood disorders - Attention-deficit/hyperactivity disorder - Anxiety disorders, obsessive-compulsive disorder, and post-traumatic stress disorder - Substance use disorders - Oppositional defiant disorder and conduct disorder - Autism spectrum disorder - Psychotic disorders - Effective teaching strategies with students who have emotional or behavioral problems - A school's mental health framework - Working with students who have mental health disorders - General education, special education, and 504 plan students - How schools are meeting the challenges of students' mental health - Summary - Appendix 1: Who diagnoses and treats child and adolescent psychiatric disorders? - Appendix 2: Comprehensive mental health evaluations - Appendix 3: The diagnostic and statistical manual of mental disorders (DSM) - Appendix 4: Overview of psychotherapy for children and adolescents - Appendix 5: Rational use of psychiatric medications.
LC Subjects	Students--Mental health.
	Students--Mental health services.
	Mentally ill children--Education.
	Emotional problems of children.
	Behavior disorders in children.
Notes	Revised edition of: The teacher's guide to student mental health. 2014.
	Includes bibliographical references and index.
Series	Norton books in education

Study guide to introductory psychiatry: a companion to the Introductory Textbook of Psychiatry, seventh edition

LCCN	2021427019
Type of material	Book
Personal name	Black, Donald W., 1956- author.

Bibliography

Main title	Study guide to introductory psychiatry: a companion to the Introductory Textbook of Psychiatry, seventh edition / Donald W. Black, M.D., Jordan Cates, M.D.
Edition	Second edition.
Published/Produced	Washington, DC: American Psychiatric Association Publishing, [2022]
Description	xi, 336 pages; 23 cm
ISBN	9781615373833 paperback
	1615373837 paperback
LC classification	RC457 .B57 2022
Related names	Cates, Jordan, author.
Summary	"Readers of the best-selling Introductory Textbook of Psychiatry, Seventh Edition--the seminal primer on the field--can now test their knowledge with this companion study guide. With a format that replicates what medical students, psychiatric residents, and others might encounter in specialty certification exams, this guide is organized along the lines of DSM-5 and features detailed questions on topics that include Diagnosis and classification Interviewing and assessment Neurobiology and genetics All DSM-5 disorders Legal issues Psychotherapy Somatic treatments Each multiple-choice question is linked to specific pages in the Textbook for ease of reference and includes plausible distractors. The answer guide includes explanations not only of the correct responses but also of why the other options are incorrect. Beyond mere rote memorization, the Study Guide to Introductory Psychiatry is designed to help learners truly assimilate and deeply encode the information in the Introductory Textbook of Psychiatry, Seventh Edition, so that they can recall it when it matters most--when speaking with the patients they treat." - Provided by publisher
Contents	Foreword - Preface - Part I: Questions - Chapter 1: Diagnosis and Classification Chapter - 2: Interviewing and Assessment - Chapter 3: Neurobiology and Genetics of Mental Illness - Chapter 4: Neurodevelopmental (Child) Disorders -

Chapter 5: Schizophrenia Spectrum and Other Psychotic Disorders - Chapter 6: Mood Disorders - Chapter 7: Anxiety Disorders - Chapter 8: Obsessive-Compulsive and Related Disorders - Chapter 9: Trauma- and Stressor-Related Disorders - Chapter 10: Somatic Symptom Disorders and Dissociative Disorders - Chapter 11: Feeding and Eating Disorders - Chapter 12: Sleep-Wake Disorders - Chapter 13: Sexual Dysfunction, Gender Dysphoria, and Paraphilic Disorders - Chapter 14: Disruptive, Impulse-Control, and Conduct Disorders - Chapter 15: Substance-Related and Addictive Disorders - Chapter 16: Neurocognitive Disorders - Chapter 17: Personality Disorders - Chapter 18: Psychiatric Emergencies - Chapter 19: Legal Issues - Chapter 20: Psychotherapy - Chapter 21: Somatic Treatments - Part II: Answer Guide - Chapter 1: Diagnosis and Classification - Chapter 2: Interviewing and Assessment - Chapter 3: Neurobiology and Genetics of Mental Illness - Chapter 4: Neurodevelopmental (Child) Disorders - Chapter 5: Schizophrenia Spectrum and Other Psychotic Disorders - Chapter 6: Mood Disorders - Chapter 7: Anxiety Disorders - Chapter 8: Obsessive-Compulsive and Related Disorders - Chapter 9: Trauma- and Stressor-Related Disorders - Chapter 10: Somatic Symptom Disorders and Dissociative Disorders - Chapter 11: Feeding and Eating Disorders - Chapter 12: Sleep-Wake Disorders - Chapter 13: Sexual Dysfunction, Gender Dysphoria, and Paraphilic Disorders - Chapter 14: Disruptive, Impulse-Control, and Conduct Disorders - Chapter 15: Substance-Related and Addictive Disorders - Chapter 16: Neurocognitive Disorders - Chapter 17: Personality Disorders - Chapter 18: Psychiatric Emergencies - Chapter 19: Legal Issues - Chapter 20: Psychotherapy - Chapter 21: Somatic Treatments.

LC Subjects	Psychiatry--Problems, exercises, etc.
Other Subjects	Mental Disorders.
	Psychiatry.

Form/Genre	Problems and exercises.

Textbook of medical psychiatry

LCCN	2019055530
Type of material	Book
Main title	Textbook of medical psychiatry / edited by Paul Summergrad, David A. Silbersweig, Philip R. Muskin, John Querques.
Edition	First edition.
Published/Produced	Washington, DC: American Psychiatric Association Publishing, [2020]
Description	xxxi, 736 pages: illustrations; 26 cm
ISBN	9781615370801 (hardcover; alk. paper) (ebook)
LC classification	RC467 .T42 2020
Related names	Summergrad, Paul, editor. Silbersweig, David, editor. Muskin, Philip R., editor. Querques, John, 1970- editor. American Psychiatric Association Publishing, issuing body.
Summary	"The Textbook of Medical Psychiatry focuses on medical disorders that can directly cause or affect the clinical presentation and course of psychiatric disorders. Clinicians who work primarily in psychiatric settings, as well as those who practice in medical settings but who have patients with co-occurring medical and psychiatric illnesses or symptoms, can benefit from a careful consideration of the medical causes of psychiatric illnesses. The editors, authorities in the field, have taken great care both in selecting the book's contributors, who are content and clinical experts, and in structuring the book for maximum learning and usefulness. The first section presents a review of approaches to diagnosis, including medical, neurological, imaging, and laboratory examination and testing. The second section provides a tour of medical disorders that can cause psychiatric symptoms or disorders, organized

Contents

by medical disease category. The third section adopts the same format as the second, offering a review of psychiatric disorders that can be caused or exacerbated by medical disorders, organized by psychiatric disorder types. The final section contains chapters on conditions that fall at the boundary between medicine and psychiatry. Even veteran clinicians may find it challenging to diagnose and treat patients who have co-occurring medical and psychiatric disorders or symptoms. The comprehensive knowledge base and clinical wisdom contained in the Textbook of Medical Psychiatry makes it the go-to resource for evaluating and managing these difficult cases"-- Provided by publisher.

An Internist's Approach to the Neuropsychiatric Patient / Joseph Rencic, M.D., Deeb Salem, M.D. - The Neurological Examination for Neuropsychiatric Assessment / Sheldon Benjamin, M.D., Margo D. Lauterbach, M.D. - The Bedside Cognitive Examination in Medical Psychiatry / Sean P. Glass, M.D. - Neuroimaging, Electroencephalography, and Lumbar Puncture in Medical Psychiatry / Daniel Talmasov, M.D., Joshua P. Klein, M.D. - Toxicological Exposures and Nutritional Deficiencies in the Psychiatric Patient / Mira Zein, M.D., M.P.H., Sharmin Khan, M.D., Jaswinder Legha, M.D., M.P.H., Lloyd Wasserman, M.D. - Cardiovascular Disease / Peter A. Shapiro, M.D. - Endocrine Disorders and Their Psychiatric Manifestations / Jane P. Gagliardi M.D., M.H.S., FACP, DFAPA - Inflammatory Diseases and Their Psychiatric Manifestations / Rolando L. Gonzalez, M.D., Charles B. Nemeroff, M.D., Ph.D. - Infectious Diseases and Their Psychiatric Manifestations / Oliver Freudenreich, M.D., Kevin M. Donnelly-Boylen, M.D., Rajesh T. Gandhi, M.D. - Gastroenterological Disease in Patients With Psychiatric Disorders / Ash Nadkarni, M.D., David

Bibliography

A. Silbersweig, M.D. - Renal Disease in Patients With Psychiatric Illness / Lily Chan, M.D., J. Michael Bostwick, M.D. - Neurological Conditions and Their Psychiatric Manifestations / Barry S. Fogel, M.D., Gaston C. Baslet, M.D., Laura T. Safar, M.D., Geoffrey S. Raynor, M.D., David A. Silbersweig, M.D. - Neurocognitive Disorders / Flannery Merideth, M.D., Ipsit V. Vahia, M.D., Dilip V. Jeste, M.D. - Neurodevelopmental Disorders / Aaron Hauptman, M.D., Sheldon Benjamin, M.D. - Cancer: Psychiatric Care of the Oncology Patient / Carlos G. Fernandez-Robles, M.D., Sean P. Glass, M.D. - Dermatology: Psychiatric Considerations in the Medical Setting. / Katherine Taylor, M.D., Janna Gordon-Elliott, M.D., Philip R. Muskin, M.D., M.A. - Obstetrics and Gynecology: Women's Mental Health and Reproductive Psychiatry / Marcela Almeida, M.D., Kara Brown, M.D., Leena Mittal, M.D., Margo Nathan, M.D., Hadine Joffe, M.D., M.Sc. - Mood Disorders Due to Medical Illnesses / Sivan Mauer, M.D., M.S. - John Querques, M.D., Paul Summergrad, M.D., - Psychotic Disorders Due to Medical Illnesses / Hannah E. Brown, M.D., Shibani Mukerji, M.D., Ph.D., Oliver Freudenreich, M.D. - Anxiety and Related Disorders: Manifestations in the General Medical Setting / Charles Hebert, M.D., David Banayan, M.D., Fernando Espi-Forcen, M.D., Ph.D., Kathryn Perticone, A.P.N., Sameera Guttikonda, M.D., Mark Pollack, M.D. - Catatonia in the Medically Ill Patient / Scott R. Beach, M.D., Gregory L. Fricchione, M.D. - Substance Use Disorders in the Medical Setting / Samata R. Sharma, M.D., Saria El Haddad, M.D., Joji Suzuki, M.D. - Chronic Pain. / Robert M. McCarron, D.O., Samir J. Sheth, M.D., Charles De Mesa, D.O. M.P.H., Michelle Burke Parish, Ph.D., M.A. - Insomnia / Karl Doghramji, M.D. - Somatic Symptom and Related Disorders / Anna L. Dickerman, M.D., Philip R. Muskin, M.D., M.A.

Other Subjects	Mental Disorders
	Comorbidity
Notes	Includes bibliographical references and index.
Additional formats	Online version: Textbook of medical psychiatry First edition. Washington, DC: American Psychiatric Association Publishing, [2020]. 9781615372829 (DLC) 2019055531

Textbook of medical psychiatry

LCCN	2019055531
Type of material	Book
Main title	Textbook of medical psychiatry / edited by Paul Summergrad, David A. Silbersweig, Philip R. Muskin, John Querques.
Edition	First edition.
Published/Produced	Washington, DC: American Psychiatric Association Publishing, [2020]
Description	1 online resource
ISBN	9781615372829 (ebook)
	(hardcover; alk. paper)
LC classification	RC467
Related names	Summergrad, Paul, editor.
	Silbersweig, David, editor.
	Muskin, Philip R., editor.
	Querques, John, 1970- editor.
	American Psychiatric Association Publishing, issuing body.
Summary	"The Textbook of Medical Psychiatry focuses on medical disorders that can directly cause or affect the clinical presentation and course of psychiatric disorders. Clinicians who work primarily in psychiatric settings, as well as those who practice in medical settings but who have patients with co-occurring medical and psychiatric illnesses or symptoms, can benefit from a careful consideration of the medical causes of psychiatric illnesses. The editors, authorities in the field, have taken great care both in selecting the book's contributors, who are content and clinical experts, and in structuring the

Contents

book for maximum learning and usefulness. The first section presents a review of approaches to diagnosis, including medical, neurological, imaging, and laboratory examination and testing. The second section provides a tour of medical disorders that can cause psychiatric symptoms or disorders, organized by medical disease category. The third section adopts the same format as the second, offering a review of psychiatric disorders that can be caused or exacerbated by medical disorders, organized by psychiatric disorder types. The final section contains chapters on conditions that fall at the boundary between medicine and psychiatry. Even veteran clinicians may find it challenging to diagnose and treat patients who have co-occurring medical and psychiatric disorders or symptoms. The comprehensive knowledge base and clinical wisdom contained in the Textbook of Medical Psychiatry makes it the go-to resource for evaluating and managing these difficult cases"-- Provided by publisher.

An Internist's Approach to the Neuropsychiatric Patient / Joseph Rencic, M.D., Deeb Salem, M.D. - The Neurological Examination for Neuropsychiatric Assessment / Sheldon Benjamin, M.D., Margo D. Lauterbach, M.D. - The Bedside Cognitive Examination in Medical Psychiatry / Sean P. Glass, M.D. - Neuroimaging, Electroencephalography, and Lumbar Puncture in Medical Psychiatry / Daniel Talmasov, M.D., Joshua P. Klein, M.D. - Toxicological Exposures and Nutritional Deficiencies in the Psychiatric Patient / Mira Zein, M.D., M.P.H., Sharmin Khan, M.D., Jaswinder Legha, M.D., M.P.H., Lloyd Wasserman, M.D. - Cardiovascular Disease / Peter A. Shapiro, M.D. - Endocrine Disorders and Their Psychiatric Manifestations / Jane P. Gagliardi M.D., M.H.S., FACP, DFAPA - Inflammatory Diseases and Their Psychiatric Manifestations / Rolando L. Gonzalez,

M.D., Charles B. Nemeroff, M.D., Ph.D. - Infectious Diseases and Their Psychiatric Manifestations / Oliver Freudenreich, M.D., Kevin M. Donnelly-Boylen, M.D., Rajesh T. Gandhi, M.D. - Gastroentcrological Disease in Patients With Psychiatric Disorders / Ash Nadkarni, M.D., David A. Silbersweig, M.D. - Renal Disease in Patients With Psychiatric Illness / Lily Chan, M.D., J. Michael Bostwick, M.D. - Neurological Conditions and Their Psychiatric Manifestations / Barry S. Fogel, M.D., Gaston C. Baslet, M.D., Laura T. Safar, M.D., Geoffrey S. Raynor, M.D., David A. Silbersweig, M.D. - Neurocognitive Disorders / Flannery Merideth, M.D., Ipsit V. Vahia, M.D., Dilip V. Jeste, M.D. - Neurodevelopmental Disorders / Aaron Hauptman, M.D., Sheldon Benjamin, M.D. - Cancer: Psychiatric Care of the Oncology Patient / Carlos G. Fernandez-Robles, M.D., Sean P. Glass, M.D. - Dermatology: Psychiatric Considerations in the Medical Setting. / Katherine Taylor, M.D., Janna Gordon-Elliott, M.D., Philip R. Muskin, M.D., M.A. - Obstetrics and Gynecology: Women's Mental Health and Reproductive Psychiatry / Marcela Almeida, M.D., Kara Brown, M.D., Leena Mittal, M.D., Margo Nathan, M.D., Hadine Joffe, M.D., M.Sc. - Mood Disorders Due to Medical Illnesses / Sivan Mauer, M.D., M.S. - John Querques, M.D., Paul Summergrad, M.D., - Psychotic Disorders Due to Medical Illnesses / Hannah E. Brown, M.D., Shibani Mukerji, M.D., Ph.D., Oliver Freudenreich, M.D. - Anxiety and Related Disorders: Manifestations in the General Medical Setting / Charles Hebert, M.D., David Banayan, M.D., Fernando Espi-Forcen, M.D., Ph.D., Kathryn Perticone, A.P.N., Sameera Guttikonda, M.D., Mark Pollack, M.D. - Catatonia in the Medically Ill Patient / Scott R. Beach, M.D., Gregory L. Fricchione, M.D. - Substance Use Disorders in the Medical Setting / Samata R. Sharma, M.D., Saria El Haddad, M.D., Joji

	Suzuki, M.D. - Chronic Pain. / Robert M. McCarron, D.O., Samir J. Sheth, M.D., Charles De Mesa, D.O. M.P.H., Michelle Burke Parish, Ph.D., M.A. - Insomnia / Karl Doghramji, M.D. - Somatic Symptom and Related Disorders / Anna L. Dickerman, M.D., Philip R. Muskin, M.D., M.A.
Other Subjects	Mental Disorders
	Comorbidity
Notes	Includes bibliographical references and index.
Additional formats	Print version: Textbook of medical psychiatry First edition. Washington, DC: American Psychiatric Association Publishing, [2020] 9781615370801 (DLC) 2019055530

The American Psychiatric Association Publishing textbook of schizophrenia

LCCN	2019045877
Type of material	Book
Uniform title	American Psychiatric Publishing textbook of schizophrenia
Main title	The American Psychiatric Association Publishing textbook of schizophrenia / edited by Jeffrey A. Lieberman, T. Scott Stroup, Diana O. Perkins, Lisa B. Dixon.
Edition	Second edition.
Published/Produced	Washington, D.C.: American Psychiatric Association Publishing, [2020]
Description	xiv, 306 pages: illustrations; 26 cm
ISBN	9781615371723 (hardcover; alk. paper)
	(epub)
LC classification	RC514 .A632 2020
Variant title	Textbook of schizophrenia
Related names	Lieberman, Jeffrey A., 1948- editor.
	Stroup, T. Scott, 1960- editor.
	Perkins, Diana O., 1958- editor.
	Dixon, Lisa B., editor.
	American Psychiatric Association, issuing body.
Summary	"Schizophrenia remains the most challenging of mental disorders confronted by psychiatrists and

	other mental health providers. Its primary manifestations-psychotic symptoms and cognitive impairment-profoundly affect the functioning of individuals with schizophrenia. This is an updated textbook covering the current state of knowledge about schizophrenia, including its causes, nature, presentation, and treatment. Chapters are written by a roster of experts in "-- Provided by publisher.
Contents	Epidemiology / Bernardo Ng, Stephanie Martinez, Steve Koh, Mauricio Tohen, James E. Gangwisch - Natural History / Diana O. Perkins, Jeffrey A. Lieberman - Psychopathology / Ryan E. Lawrence, Michael B. First - Cultural Variations of Psychotic Disorders / Neil Krishan Aggarwal, Roberto Lewis-Fernández - Causes / Matcheri S. Keshavan, Paulo L. Lizano, Seth W. Perry, Konasale M. Prasad, Julio Licinio - Pathophysiological Theories / Donald C. Goff - Neurobiology / L. Fredrik Jarskog, T. Wilson Woo - Pharmacologic and Somatic Therapies / T. Scott Stroup, Diana O. Perkins, Daniel C. Javitt - Psychosocial and Rehabilitative Therapies / Alice Medalia, Alice Saperstein, Paul Grant - Co-occurring Disorders and Conditions / Sarah Pratt, Melanie Bennett, Mary F. Brunette - Evidence-Based Models of Service Delivery / Michael T. Compton, Marc W. Manseau - Person- and Family-Centered Care / Nev Jones, Lisa Dixon
Other Subjects	Schizophrenia
Notes	Preceded by The American Psychiatric Publishing textbook of schizophrenia / edited by edited by Jeffrey A. Lieberman, T. Scott Stroup, Diana O. Perkins. 1st ed. c2006. Includes bibliographical references and index.
Additional formats	Online version: The American Psychiatric Association publishing textbook of schizophrenia Second. Washington, D.C.: American Psychiatric Association Publishing, 2020. 9781615372911 (DLC) 2019045878

The American Psychiatric Association Publishing textbook of schizophrenia	
LCCN	2019045878
Type of material	Book
Uniform title	American Psychiatric Publishing textbook of schizophrenia
Main title	The American Psychiatric Association Publishing textbook of schizophrenia / edited by Jeffrey A. Lieberman, M.D., T. Scott Stroup, M.D., M.P.H, Diana O. Perkins, M.D., M.P.H., Lisa B. Dixon, M.D., M.P.H..
Edition	Second edition.
Published/Produced	Washington, D.C.: American Psychiatric Association Publishing, [2020]
Description	1 online resource
ISBN	9781615372911 (epub)
	(hardcover; alk. paper)
LC classification	RC514
Variant title	Textbook of schizophrenia
Related names	Lieberman, Jeffrey A., 1948- editor.
	Stroup, T. Scott, 1960- editor.
	Perkins, Diana O., 1958- editor.
	Dixon, Lisa B., editor.
	American Psychiatric Association, issuing body.
Summary	"Schizophrenia remains the most challenging of mental disorders confronted by psychiatrists and other mental health providers. Its primary manifestations-psychotic symptoms and cognitive impairment-profoundly affect the functioning of individuals with schizophrenia. This is an updated textbook covering the current state of knowledge about schizophrenia, including its causes, nature, presentation, and treatment. Chapters are written by a roster of experts in "-- Provided by publisher.
Contents	Epidemiology / Bernardo Ng, Stephanie Martinez, Steve Koh, Mauricio Tohen, James E. Gangwisch - Natural History / Diana O. Perkins, Jeffrey A. Lieberman - Psychopathology / Ryan E. Lawrence, Michael B. First - Cultural Variations of Psychotic

Bibliography 183

	Disorders / Neil Krishan Aggarwal, Roberto Lewis-Fernández - Causes / Matcheri S. Keshavan, Paulo L. Lizano, Seth W. Perry, Konasale M. Prasad, Julio Licinio - Pathophysiological Theories / Donald C. Goff - Neurobiology / L. Fredrik Jarskog, T. Wilson Woo - Pharmacologic and Somatic Therapies / T. Scott Stroup, Diana O. Perkins, Daniel C. Javitt - Psychosocial and Rehabilitative Therapies / Alice Medalia, Alice Saperstein, Paul Grant - Co-occurring Disorders and Conditions / Sarah Pratt, Melanie Bennett, Mary F. Brunette - Evidence-Based Models of Service Delivery / Michael T. Compton, Marc W. Manseau - Person- and Family-Centered Care / Nev Jones, Lisa Dixon
Other Subjects	Schizophrenia
Notes	Preceded by The American Psychiatric Publishing textbook of schizophrenia / edited by edited by Jeffrey A. Lieberman, T. Scott Stroup, Diana O. Perkins. 1st ed. c2006.
	Includes bibliographical references and index.
Additional formats	Print version: American Psychiatric Publishing textbook of schizophrenia The American Psychiatric Association Publishing textbook of schizophrenia Second edition. Washington, D.C.: American Psychiatric Association Publishing, [2020] 9781615371723 (DLC) 2019045877

The clinical use of antipsychotic plasma levels

LCCN	2021012649
Type of material	Book
Personal name	Meyer, Jonathan M., 1962- author.
Main title	The clinical use of antipsychotic plasma levels / Jonathan M Meyer, Stephen M Stahl; with illustrations by Nancy Munter.
Published/Produced	Cambridge; New York, NY: Cambridge University Press, 2021.
Description	1 online resource
ISBN	9781009002103 (ebook)
	(paperback)

184   Bibliography

LC classification	RM333.5
Related names	Stahl, Stephen M., 1951- author.
Summary	"The use of antipsychotics to treat schizophrenia is fraught with many layers of complexity, as prescribers try to tailor the pharmacodynamic properties of an agent to a specific patient based primarily on subjective response. Variations in drug metabolism related to genetic polymorphisms, or to medication or environmental exposures (e.g., smoking), and variable adherence with oral medications lead to scenarios that confound even seasoned clinicians. Excluding the realization that up to one-third of schizophrenia patients may not respond adequately to non-clozapine antipsychotics, 60 years of antipsychotic research has demonstrated that dose is a poor correlate of response likelihood, whereas plasma drug levels represent the best clinically available tool that quantifies the relationship between drug exposure and central nervous system (CNS) activity.[1] The classic equation by psychopharmacologist Sheldon Preskorn illustrates the variables involved in clinical drug response (Figure 1.1)"-- Provided by publisher.
Contents	Sampling times for oral and long acting injectable agents - The therapeutic threshold and the point of futility - Level interpretation including laboratory reporting issues, responding to high plasma issues, responding to high plasma levels, special situations (hepatic dysfunction, renal dysfunction and hemodialysis, bariatric surgery) - Tracking oral antipsychotic adherence - What is an adequate antipsychotic trial-using plasma levels to optimize psychiatric response and tolerability - Important concepts about first generation antipsychotics - Haloperidol and haloperidol decanoate - Fluphenazine and fluphenazine decanoate - Perphenazine and perphenazine decanoate - Zuclopenthixol and zuclopenthixol decanoate; flupenthixol and flupenthixol decanoate -

	Chlorpromazine, loxapine, thiothixene, trifluoperazine - Important concepts about second generation antipsychotics - Clozapine - Risperidone oral and long acting injectable, paliperidone oral and long acting injectable - Olanzapine and olanzapine pamoate - Aripiprazole, aripiprazole monohydrate and aripiprazole lauroxil - Amisulpride, asenapine, lurasidone, brexpiprazole, cariprazine.
Other Subjects	Antipsychotic Agents--blood
	Dose-Response Relationship, Drug
	Antipsychotic Agents--therapeutic use
	Dose-Response Relationship, Drug
	Psychotic Disorders--drug therapy
	Schizophrenia--drug therapy
	Medical / Mental Health
	Medical / Mental Health
Notes	Includes bibliographical references and index.
Additional formats	Print version: Meyer, Jonathan M., 1962- The clinical use of antipsychotic plasma levels Cambridge; New York, NY: Cambridge University Press, 2021. 9781009009898 (DLC) 2021012648
Series	Stahl's handbooks
	Stahl's handbooks.

The clinical use of antipsychotic plasma levels

LCCN	2021012648
Type of material	Book
Personal name	Meyer, Jonathan M., 1962- author.
Main title	The clinical use of antipsychotic plasma levels / Jonathan M Meyer, Stephen M Stahl; with illustrations by Nancy Munter.
Published/Produced	Cambridge; New York, NY: Cambridge University Press, 2021.
ISBN	9781009009898 (paperback)
	(ebook)
LC classification	RM333.5
Related names	Stahl, Stephen M., 1951- author.
Summary	"The use of antipsychotics to treat schizophrenia is fraught with many layers of complexity, as

Contents

prescribers try to tailor the pharmacodynamic properties of an agent to a specific patient based primarily on subjective response. Variations in drug metabolism related to genetic polymorphisms, or to medication or environmental exposures (e.g., smoking), and variable adherence with oral medications lead to scenarios that confound even seasoned clinicians. Excluding the realization that up to one-third of schizophrenia patients may not respond adequately to non-clozapine antipsychotics, 60 years of antipsychotic research has demonstrated that dose is a poor correlate of response likelihood, whereas plasma drug levels represent the best clinically available tool that quantifies the relationship between drug exposure and central nervous system (CNS) activity.[1] The classic equation by psychopharmacologist Sheldon Preskorn illustrates the variables involved in clinical drug response (Figure 1.1)"-- Provided by publisher. Sampling times for oral and long acting injectable agents - The therapeutic threshold and the point of futility - Level interpretation including laboratory reporting issues, responding to high plasma issues, responding to high plasma levels, special situations (hepatic dysfunction, renal dysfunction and hemodialysis, bariatric surgery) - Tracking oral antipsychotic adherence - What is an adequate antipsychotic trial-using plasma levels to optimize psychiatric response and tolerability - Important concepts about first generation antipsychotics - Haloperidol and haloperidol decanoate - Fluphenazine and fluphenazine decanoate - Perphenazine and perphenazine decanoate - Zuclopenthixol and zuclopenthixol decanoate; flupenthixol and flupenthixol decanoate - Chlorpromazine, loxapine, thiothixene, trifluoperazine - Important concepts about second generation antipsychotics - Clozapine - Risperidone oral and long acting injectable, paliperidone oral and

	long acting injectable - Olanzapine and olanzapine pamoate - Aripiprazole, aripiprazole monohydrate and aripiprazole lauroxil - Amisulpride, asenapine, lurasidone, brexpiprazole, cariprazine.
Other Subjects	Antipsychotic Agents--blood
	Dose-Response Relationship, Drug
	Antipsychotic Agents--therapeutic use
	Dose-Response Relationship, Drug
	Psychotic Disorders--drug therapy
	Schizophrenia--drug therapy
	Medical / Mental Health
	Medical / Mental Health
Notes	Includes bibliographical references and index.
Additional formats	Online version: Meyer, Jonathan M, 1962- The clinical use of antipsychotic plasma levels Cambridge; New York, NY: Cambridge University Press, 2021 9781009002103 (DLC) 2021012649
Series	Stahl's handbooks
	Stahl's handbooks.

The dialectical behavior therapy skills workbook for psychosis: manage your emotions, reduce symptoms, and get back to your life

LCCN	2020034747
Type of material	Book
Personal name	Mullen, Maggie, author.
Main title	The dialectical behavior therapy skills workbook for psychosis: manage your emotions, reduce symptoms, and get back to your life / Maggie Mullen, LCSW.
Published/Produced	Oakland: New Harbinger Publications, Inc., 2021.
Description	1 online resource.
ISBN	9781684036608 (epub)
	9781684036592 (pdf)
	(trade paperback)
LC classification	RC512
Summary	"People with psychotic spectrum disorders often struggle with paranoia, auditory hallucinations, poor concentration and memory, and emotional dysregulation. Unfortunately, there are very limited resources available to them, outside of therapy. At

	long last, The Dialectical Behavior Therapy Skills Workbook for Psychosis teaches readers powerful and evidence-based skills to help them manage their emotions and reduce symptoms so they can get back to living their lives"-- Provided by publisher.
LC Subjects	Psychoses--Treatment.
	Dialectical behavior therapy.
Notes	Includes bibliographical references.
Additional formats	Print version: Mullen, Maggie. The dialectical behavior therapy skills workbook for psychosis Oakland: New Harbinger Publications, 2021. 9781684036431 (DLC) 2020034746

The dialectical behavior therapy skills workbook for psychosis: manage your emotions, reduce symptoms, and get back to your life

LCCN	2020034746
Type of material	Book
Personal name	Mullen, Maggie, author.
Main title	The dialectical behavior therapy skills workbook for psychosis: manage your emotions, reduce symptoms, and get back to your life / Maggie Mullen, LCSW, Douglas Turkington.
Published/Produced	Oakland: New Harbinger Publications, 2021.
ISBN	9781684036431 (trade paperback)
	(pdf)
	(epub)
LC classification	RC512 .M85 2021
Related names	Turkington, Douglas, author.
Summary	"People with psychotic spectrum disorders often struggle with paranoia, auditory hallucinations, poor concentration and memory, and emotional dysregulation. Unfortunately, there are very limited resources available to them, outside of therapy. At long last, The Dialectical Behavior Therapy Skills Workbook for Psychosis teaches readers powerful and evidence-based skills to help them manage their emotions and reduce symptoms so they can get back to living their lives"-- Provided by publisher.
LC Subjects	Psychoses--Treatment.

	Dialectical behavior therapy.
Notes	Includes bibliographical references.
Additional formats	Online version: Mullen, Maggie, The dialectical behavior therapy skills workbook for psychosis Oakland: New Harbinger Publications, 2021. 9781684036592 (DLC) 2020034747

The first episode of psychosis: a guide for young people and their families

LCCN	2020026339
Type of material	Book
Personal name	Compton, Michael T., author.
Main title	The first episode of psychosis: a guide for young people and their families / Beth Broussard, Michael T. Compton.
Edition	Second edition.
Published/Produced	New York, NY: Oxford University Press, [2021]
Description	1 online resource
ISBN	9780197542514
	9780190920708 (epub)
	(paperback)
LC classification	RC512
Related names	Broussard, Beth, author.
Summary	"Now in its second edition, The First Episode of Psychosis is the ideal book for young people and their families experiencing the frightening and confusing initial episode of psychosis, which often occurs during late adolescence or early adulthood. The updated edition includes information on specialized early intervention services, going back to school and work, and the latest treatments and medicines. The book covers a range of topics essential for young people and families facing the challenges of psychosis. Topics covered include early warning signs, symptoms, types of primary psychotic disorders such as schizophrenia and schizophreniform disorder, evaluation, treatment, and healthy lifestyle choices. Worksheets helps readers to track and better understand their own experiences, and to openly communicate with care

	providers. An extensive glossary clarifies the dizzying array of terms used by medical professionals. Optimistic, practical, and recovery-oriented, The First Episode of Psychosis will help young people and their families take an active, informed role in their care as they take steps towards achieving their goals"-- Provided by publisher.
Contents	What Is Psychosis? - What Are the Symptoms of Psychosis? - What Diagnoses Are Associated with Psychosis? - What Causes Primary Psychotic Disorders Like Schizophrenia? - Finding the Best Care: Specialty Programs for Early Psychosis - The Initial Evaluation of Psychosis - Medicines Used to Treat Psychosis - Psychosocial Treatments for Early Psychosis - Follow-Up and Sticking with Treatment - Early Warning Signs and Preventing a Relapse - Staying Healthy - Embracing Recovery - Going Back to School and Work - Reducing Stress, Coping, and Communicating Effectively: Tips for Family Members and Young People with Psychosis - Understanding Mental Health First Aid for Psychosis.
LC Subjects	Psychoses--Popular works.
Notes	Michael T. Compton appears as the first named author on the earlier edition.
	Includes bibliographical references and index.
Additional formats	Print version: Compton, Michael T.. The first episode of psychosis Second edition. New York, NY: Oxford University Press, [2021] 9780190920685 (DLC) 2020026338

The first episode of psychosis: a guide for young people and their families

LCCN	2020026338
Type of material	Book
Personal name	Compton, Michael T., author.
Main title	The first episode of psychosis: a guide for young people and their families / Beth Broussard, Michael T. Compton.
Edition	Second edition.

Published/Produced	New York, NY: Oxford University Press, [2021]
ISBN	9780190920685 (paperback)
	(epub)
LC classification	RC512 .C58 2021
Related names	Broussard, Beth, author.
Summary	"Now in its second edition, The First Episode of Psychosis is the ideal book for young people and their families experiencing the frightening and confusing initial episode of psychosis, which often occurs during late adolescence or early adulthood. The updated edition includes information on specialized early intervention services, going back to school and work, and the latest treatments and medicines. The book covers a range of topics essential for young people and families facing the challenges of psychosis. Topics covered include early warning signs, symptoms, types of primary psychotic disorders such as schizophrenia and schizophreniform disorder, evaluation, treatment, and healthy lifestyle choices. Worksheets helps readers to track and better understand their own experiences, and to openly communicate with care providers. An extensive glossary clarifies the dizzying array of terms used by medical professionals. Optimistic, practical, and recovery-oriented, The First Episode of Psychosis will help young people and their families take an active, informed role in their care as they take steps towards achieving their goals"-- Provided by publisher.
Contents	What Is Psychosis? - What Are the Symptoms of Psychosis? - What Diagnoses Are Associated with Psychosis? - What Causes Primary Psychotic Disorders Like Schizophrenia? - Finding the Best Care: Specialty Programs for Early Psychosis - The Initial Evaluation of Psychosis - Medicines Used to Treat Psychosis - Psychosocial Treatments for Early Psychosis - Follow-Up and Sticking with Treatment - Early Warning Signs and Preventing a Relapse - Staying Healthy - Embracing Recovery - Going Back

	to School and Work - Reducing Stress, Coping, and Communicating Effectively: Tips for Family Members and Young People with Psychosis - Understanding Mental Health First Aid for Psychosis.
LC Subjects	Psychoses--Popular works.
Notes	Michael T. Compton appears as the first named author on the earlier edition.
	Includes bibliographical references and index.
Additional formats	Online version: Compton, Michael T. First episode of psychosis Second edition. New York, NY: Oxford University Press, [2021] 9780190920708 (DLC) 2020026339

The Maudsley guidelines on advanced prescribing in psychosis

LCCN	2019047708
Type of material	Book
Personal name	Morrison, Paul, 1956- author.
Main title	The Maudsley guidelines on advanced prescribing in psychosis / Paul Morrison, David M. Taylor, Phillip McGuire.
Published/Produced	Hoboken, NJ: Wiley-Blackwell, 2020.
Description	1 online resource
ISBN	9781119578437 (epub)
	9781119578529 (adobe pdf)
	(paperback)
LC classification	RC483
Variant title	Guidelines on advanced prescribing in psychosis
Related names	Taylor, David, 1963- author.
	McGuire, Philip, author.
Summary	"The goal for this text is to emphasize that treatment of psychosis must be tailored to the needs of individual patients. While a given diagnosis may suggest principle mechanisms under prescription guidelines, standard treatment of psychosis is unfeasible due to no two patients suffering from an identical illness. This text therefore aims to contrast the one-size-fits-all treatment that general medicine has taken for granted, and instead focuses on building

Contents	psychiatrist and patient relationships to foster individual treatment plans"-- Provided by publisher. Psychosis - Towards evidence based treatments for psychosis - The antipsychotics - Bipolar disorder - The role of talking therapies in the treatment of psychosis - Side effects of antipsychotic treatment - Services: pathway specific care - Measuring outcomes.
Other Subjects	Psychotic Disorders--drug therapy Antipsychotic Agents--side effects Evidence-Based Medicine Physician-Patient Relations Treatment Outcome
Notes	Includes bibliographical references and index.
Additional formats	Print version: Morrison, Paul, 1956- Maudsley guidelines on advanced prescribing in psychosis Hoboken, NJ: Wiley-Blackwell, 2020 9781119578444 (DLC) 2019047707

The Maudsley guidelines on advanced prescribing in psychosis

LCCN	2019047707
Type of material	Book
Personal name	Morrison, Paul, 1956- author.
Main title	The Maudsley guidelines on advanced prescribing in psychosis / Paul Morrison, David M. Taylor, Phillip McGuire.
Published/Produced	Hoboken, NJ: Wiley-Blackwell, 2020.
ISBN	9781119578444 (paperback) (adobe pdf) (epub)
LC classification	RC483
Variant title	Guidelines on advanced prescribing in psychosis
Related names	Taylor, David, 1963- author. McGuire, Philip, author.
Summary	"The goal for this text is to emphasize that treatment of psychosis must be tailored to the needs of individual patients. While a given diagnosis may suggest principle mechanisms under prescription guidelines, standard treatment of psychosis is

	unfeasible due to no two patients suffering from an identical illness. This text therefore aims to contrast the one-size-fits-all treatment that general medicine has taken for granted, and instead focuses on building psychiatrist and patient relationships to foster individual treatment plans"-- Provided by publisher.
Contents	Psychosis - Towards evidence based treatments for psychosis - The antipsychotics - Bipolar disorder - The role of talking therapies in the treatment of psychosis - Side effects of antipsychotic treatment - Services: pathway specific care - Measuring outcomes.
Other Subjects	Psychotic Disorders--drug therapy Antipsychotic Agents--side effects Evidence-Based Medicine Physician-Patient Relations Treatment Outcome
Notes	Includes bibliographical references and index.
Additional formats	Online version: Morrison, Paul, 1956- Maudsley guidelines on advanced prescribing in psychosis Hoboken, NJ: Wiley-Blackwell, 2020 9781119578437 (DLC) 2019047708

The Oxford handbook of autism and co-occurring psychiatric conditions

LCCN	2020933023
Type of material	Book
Main title	The Oxford handbook of autism and co-occurring psychiatric conditions / edited by Susan W. White, Brenna B. Maddox, and Carla A. Mazefsky.
Published/Produced	New York, NY: Oxford University Press, 2020.
Description	xxvi, 443 pages: illustrations; 27 cm
ISBN	9780190910761 (hardcover) 0190910763 (hardcover)
LC classification	RC553.A88 O94 2020
Variant title	Handbook of autism and co-occurring psychiatric conditions
Related names	White, Susan Williams, editor. Maddox, Brenna B., editor. Mazefsky, Carla A., editor.

Summary

Co-occurring psychiatric conditions are extremely common among people who have autism spectrum disorder (ASD). The Oxford Handbook of Autism and Co-Occurring Psychiatric Conditions presents a compilation of the latest research in this area, summarized by internationally renowned experts. Each chapter presents an overview of the problem or disorder including information on prevalence in ASD and in the general public and a synthesis of the research on etiology, diagnostic best practices, and evidence-based intervention approaches. Case studies bring these concepts to life, and each chapter concludes with suggestions for future research directions in order to further develop our scientific and clinical understanding of the particular comorbidity. Given the fact that comorbidity is often a chronic and pervasive concern, this Handbook takes a lifespan approach, with each chapter touching on developmental aspects of the targeted problem, from early childhood through adulthood. The concluding section of the Handbook is comprised of content on clinical considerations and research approaches, including chapters on medications commonly used to treat co-occurring conditions, strategies for managing crisis situations in this clinical population, and community partnerships within an implementation science framework.

Contents

Foreword / John Elder Robison - Part I: Overview 1. Autism Spectrum Disorder and co-occurring psychiatric conditions: a conceptual framework / Virginia Carter Leno and Emily Simonoff - Part II: Co-occurring conditions - Co-occurring mood problems in Autism Spectrum Disorder / Katherine Gotham, Florencia Pezzimenti, Mareike Eydt-Beebe, Gloria T. Han, and Catherine G. Herrington - Schizophrenia and other psychotic disorders in Autism Spectrum Disorder / Jennifer H. Foss-Feig, Stacey Lurie, and Maya F. Hubert - Autism spectrum disorder and co-occurring addiction / Patricia J. M.

van Wijngaarden-Cremers - Anxiety in Autism Spectrum Disorder: a case of blurred boundaries / Lawrence Scahill and Andrea N. Evans - Obsessive-compulsive and related disorders in Autism Spectrum Disorder / Katelyn M. Dyason, Sharna L. Mathieu, Donna L. Griffiths, and Lara J. Farrell - Post-traumatic Stress Disorder in individuals with Autism Spectrum Disorder / Connor M. Kerns, Chandler Puhy, Chelsea M. Day, and Steven J. Berkowitz - Oppositional Defiant Disorder and related disruptive behaviors in Autism Spectrum Disorder / Karen Bearss and Aaron Kaat - Attention Deficit Hyperactivity Disorder in Autism Spectrum Disorder: a high-risk co-occurring condition / Benjamin E. Yerys - Intellectual disability in Autism Spectrum Disorder / Jill C. Fodstad, Rebecca Elias, and Shivali Sarawgi - Co-occurrence of autism and gender diversity / John F. Strang, Dana L. Rofey, and Eleonora Sadikova - Part III: Related problems - Psychosexual problems, sexual deviance and promoting sexual health in autistic adolescents and adults / Kirstin Greaves-Lord, Jeroen Dewinter, Lennart Pedersen, Olive Healy, and Mark A. Stokes - Eating issues in Autism Spectrum Disorder / Emily S. Kuschner and Gregory L. Wallace - Sleep problems in Autism Spectrum Disorder / Margaret C. Souders, Briana J. Taylor, and Stefanie Zavodny Jackson - Aggression in Autism Spectrum Disorder / Micah O. Mazurek - Understanding executive function challenges in Autism Spectrum Disorders / Cara E. Pugliese, Gregory L. Wallace, Laura Gutermuth Anthony, and Lauren Kenworthy - Self-injurious behavior in individuals with Autism Spectrum Disorder / Jennifer N. Haddock and Louis P. Hagopian - Suicidality and self-harm in Autism Spectrum conditions / Sarah Cassidy - Part 4: Current clinical practices and promising research approaches - Medications to treat co-occurring psychiatric conditions in Autism Spectrum Disorder / Bryan H.

	King, Agnieszka Rynkiewicz, Malgorzata Janas-Kozik, and Marta Tyszkewicz-Nwafor - Model for addressing crisis behavior in youth with Autism Spectrum Disorder within a functional and contextual framework / Robin L. Gabriels and Julia Barnes - Designing Autism Spectrum Disorder interventions for community implementation: addressing children's challenging behaviors in publicly-funded mental health services / Lauren Brookman-Frazee, Amy Drahota, Colby Chlebowski, Yael Koenig, Katherine Nguyen Williams, Barry Hill, and Julie McPherson - Synthesis: current state of the science and future directions / Brenna B. Maddox, Carla A. Mazefsky, and Susan W. White.
LC Subjects	Autism spectrum disorders.
	Autism spectrum disorders--Case studies.
Other Subjects	Autism Spectrum Disorder--complications.
	Mental Disorders--complications.
	Evidence-Based Practice.
	Autism spectrum disorders.
	Comorbidity.
Form/Genre	Case Reports.
Notes	Includes bibliographical references and index.
Series	Oxford library of psychology
	Oxford library of psychology.

Index

A

acting out, 79, 80, 82, 83
activity(ies), 2, 3, 7, 11, 12, 16, 18, 20, 23, 25, 28, 30, 31, 39, 45, 46, 53, 63, 64, 66, 67, 69, 70, 88, 184, 186
adolescence, v, vii, viii, 61, 62, 65, 68, 70, 71, 85, 94, 106, 108, 109, 110, 155, 157, 189, 191
affective disorders, 7, 8, 11, 13, 24, 27, 30

B

behaviour, 4, 12, 17, 36, 39, 40, 43, 44, 45, 46, 47, 53, 55, 57, 63, 80, 82, 94, 95, 100, 102, 103, 104, 114, 116, 124, 126, 156, 167, 171, 187, 188, 189, 196
Bell Lysaker emotion recognition task (BLERT), viii, 35, 38, 43, 50, 51
bipolar depression, vii, 1, 2, 7, 8, 11, 12, 19, 20, 163
bipolar disorder, vii, viii, 1, 8, 25, 26, 27, 28, 29, 30, 31, 62, 99, 139, 140, 141, 148, 149, 151, 153, 162, 168, 170, 193, 194
brain, viii, 7, 8, 9, 10, 11, 12, 13, 14, 15, 16, 17, 18, 19, 20, 21, 23, 24, 25, 26, 27, 28, 29, 30, 31, 57, 61, 65, 66, 67, 72, 75, 83, 91, 92, 96, 97, 123, 125, 126, 133, 136, 138, 140, 141, 145, 147, 168, 170

C

cognition, 4, 5, 6, 9, 16, 19, 23, 28, 37, 56, 58, 73, 93, 94, 123, 125, 136, 138

cognitive social and affective impairment, 2
cognitive, social and affective (CAS), vii, 1, 5
communication(s), 8, 12, 23, 45, 47, 55, 78, 79
concept(s), vii, 1, 3, 22, 36, 39, 43, 45, 46, 47, 48, 54, 57, 62, 123, 126, 145, 146, 151, 153, 158, 159, 160, 161, 165, 166, 184, 186, 195
connection(s), 5, 10, 11, 20, 21, 36, 37, 44, 46, 47
connectivity, 9, 10, 11, 12, 13, 14, 15, 16, 17, 19, 20, 21, 22, 23, 24, 25, 26, 28, 29, 30, 31, 66, 72
contributing factors, vii, viii, 62
contribution(s), v, 1, 48, 72, 104
Cornell scale for depression in dementia (CSDD), 7
countertransference, 79, 80

D

deficit symptoms, vii, 1
dementia, vii, 1, 2, 3, 7, 22, 24, 62, 85, 91, 93, 124, 126
depression, viii, 5, 6, 7, 11, 13, 19, 20, 21, 23, 25, 26, 30, 62, 85, 99, 124, 126, 133, 139, 140, 141, 146, 147, 148, 149, 150, 158, 160, 162, 163
development, vii, viii, 8, 15, 17, 22, 23, 35, 36, 38, 43, 44, 50, 56, 59, 62, 63, 64, 65, 66, 67, 69, 70, 71, 94, 104, 115, 117, 123, 125
diagnosis, viii, 7, 12, 14, 15, 19, 21, 23, 31, 62, 63, 68, 69, 74, 78, 94, 96, 97, 101,

103, 105, 106, 108, 113, 114, 118, 119, 123, 126, 130, 132, 158, 159, 160, 161, 168, 170, 172, 174, 178, 192, 193
diagnostic and statistical manual of mental disorders (DSM-V), vii, viii, 4, 61, 63, 71, 95, 97, 115, 116, 117, 171
digit symbol substitution test (DSST), vii, 1, 6, 24, 26

E

emotion(s), viii, 4, 8, 12, 13, 29, 35, 37, 38, 39, 43, 45, 46, 47, 50, 52, 54, 82, 83, 152, 153, 187, 188
evaluation, vii, 1, 5, 23, 35, 36, 48, 50, 53, 56, 72, 92, 128, 129, 136, 138, 189, 190, 191
external, 18, 40, 52, 64, 82, 83

F

flexible thinking, 46
foundation, 2, 3, 46, 47, 154
functional magnetic resonance imaging (fMRI), vii, 1, 2, 7, 8, 11, 13, 14, 15, 17, 18, 19, 21, 23, 24, 26, 28, 30, 31
fundamental, 5, 12, 45, 46, 49, 65, 84, 122, 125

G

group therapy, v, viii, 35, 41, 44, 46, 49, 52, 56, 58, 59, 84, 127, 128, 129
group(s), v, vii, 1, 2, 3, 4, 12, 20, 21, 35, 36, 38, 39, 41, 43, 44, 45, 46, 49, 50, 52, 53, 54, 55, 56, 58, 59, 61, 63, 70, 77, 78, 79, 84, 91, 107, 127, 128, 129, 140, 141, 142, 151, 153, 157, 159, 162

H

hinting task, viii, 35, 38, 42, 50, 51

I

impairment, 5, 6, 7, 8, 10, 12, 14, 16, 17, 19, 23, 25, 28, 36, 37, 63, 64, 90, 92, 181, 182
interactional, v, viii, 35, 44, 56, 59
interactive, v, 35, 44, 45
intervention(s), v, 9, 11, 35, 37, 39, 48, 50, 57, 59, 68, 69, 71, 72, 73, 74, 79, 87, 89, 98, 101, 102, 156, 189, 191, 195, 197

M

major depressive disorder, vii, 1, 2, 11, 20, 24, 26, 27, 28, 29, 30, 31, 123, 125, 151, 153
measurement(s), 41, 50
memory, 5, 7, 9, 12, 14, 15, 16, 17, 18, 20, 23, 24, 25, 26, 29, 30, 38, 79, 83, 92, 187, 188
mental illness, viii, 2, 8, 37, 44, 62, 105, 107, 109, 110, 111, 112, 113, 115, 116, 121, 122, 127, 129, 139, 140, 141, 142, 143
mental states, 36, 38, 40, 41, 46, 47, 52
mentalization, v, viii, 35, 39, 40, 41, 43, 44, 45, 46, 47, 48, 52, 53, 54, 55, 56, 57, 58, 59, 104
mentalization-based treatment, 41, 53, 57
metacognition, viii, 35, 37, 38, 39, 43, 44, 56, 57, 58
mind(s), 7, 31, 36, 40, 41, 44, 45, 46, 47, 83, 94, 105, 107, 109, 115, 116, 166, 167
music therapists, v, vii, ix, 77, 78, 82, 83, 84, 85, 86
music therapy, ix, 77, 78, 79, 83, 84, 85, 86

N

narcissism, viii, 77, 78, 83, 84, 85
narcissistic, v, vii, viii, 77, 78, 80, 81, 82, 83, 84, 85, 86
narcissistic personality traits, ix, 78, 80, 82
narcissistic wounds, vii, ix, 77, 78, 80, 81, 82, 83, 84, 85

Index

negative, v, vii, 1, 4, 5, 8, 9, 10, 15, 16, 19, 20, 22, 23, 24, 25, 26, 27, 28, 29, 30, 31, 38, 43, 52, 57, 63, 64, 66, 72, 75, 88, 134, 135
negative syndrome scale (PANSS), 5, 16, 23

O

outcome, 2, 41, 53, 71, 89, 127, 129, 193, 194

P

patient(s), viii, ix, 5, 6, 7, 8, 9, 10, 11, 12, 13, 14, 15, 16, 17, 18, 19, 20, 21, 22, 23, 24, 25, 26, 27, 28, 29, 30, 35, 36, 37, 38, 39, 41, 43, 44, 45, 48, 49, 50, 52, 53, 54, 55, 56, 57, 58, 63, 65, 67, 72, 74, 78, 79, 80, 81, 82, 83, 84, 85, 87, 93, 94, 95, 97, 104, 120, 127, 128, 129, 134, 135, 136, 138, 144, 151, 152, 155, 158, 160, 162, 163, 172, 174, 175, 177, 178, 184, 186, 192, 193, 194
performance, 6, 7, 14, 17, 30, 36, 43, 46, 49, 65, 70, 90, 91, 151, 153
personality, v, 58, 63, 77, 81, 83, 85, 86, 91, 92, 96, 98, 99, 106, 108, 114, 118, 119, 121, 122, 131, 132, 140, 141, 142, 143, 148, 149, 150, 151, 152, 153, 155, 157, 158, 160, 173
personality wounds, v, 77
physical, 52, 79, 87, 88, 145, 146, 147, 155
positive, 5, 13, 15, 16, 20, 23, 25, 38, 39, 41, 43, 44, 46, 53, 57, 63, 64, 67, 69, 71, 72, 134, 135
prevention, 68, 69, 73, 78, 101, 148, 149, 150, 155
prognosis, v, viii, 1, 4, 62, 68, 69, 71, 73, 148, 149
program(s), vii, 36, 39, 41, 43, 44, 50, 53, 56, 59, 158, 160
proof of concept (PoC), v, vii, 35, 36, 48, 56
propriety, v, vii, 35, 36

psychosis, v, vii, viii, 1, 2, 4, 13, 22, 27, 40, 41, 48, 57, 58, 62, 63, 65, 66, 67, 68, 69, 71, 72, 73, 74, 75, 87, 88, 104, 127, 128, 129, 144, 148, 150, 162, 187, 188, 189, 190, 191, 192, 193, 194
psychotic disorders, v, vii, viii, 57, 59, 61, 62, 63, 64, 66, 67, 68, 69, 71, 88, 89, 90, 94, 96, 97, 100, 102, 105, 106, 108, 109, 110, 111, 112, 114, 118, 119, 120, 124, 126, 128, 129, 130, 132, 133, 134, 135, 136, 137, 138, 144, 146, 147, 148, 149, 151, 153, 155, 157, 164, 165, 166, 167, 168, 170, 171, 173, 176, 179, 181, 183, 185, 187, 189, 190, 191, 193, 194, 195

S

schizophrenia, v, vii, viii, 1, 2, 3, 4, 5, 7, 8, 9, 10, 11, 12, 14, 15, 16, 17, 18, 19, 22, 23, 24, 25, 26, 27, 28, 29, 30, 31, 35, 36, 37, 38, 39, 41, 43, 44, 50, 53, 55, 56, 57, 58, 59, 61, 62, 63, 66, 72, 73, 74, 88, 94, 100, 114, 120, 123, 125, 130, 132, 134, 135,137, 138, 139, 151, 153, 155, 157, 162, 163, 165, 166, 168, 170, 173, 180, 181, 182, 183, 184, 185, 187, 189, 190, 191, 195
self-reflection, 37, 39, 45, 46, 47
social, v, viii, 4, 9, 14, 24, 26, 28, 29, 35, 36, 37, 38, 39, 40, 41, 43, 44, 45, 47, 48, 50, 54, 55, 56, 57, 58, 59, 63, 64, 65, 68, 69, 70, 71, 74, 79, 83, 87, 88, 99, 101, 113, 115, 117, 151, 153, 154, 164, 168, 169, 170
social cognition, v, viii, 26, 28, 35, 37, 38, 39, 41, 43, 44, 50, 56, 57, 58, 59, 88
social thinking, 39, 41, 56, 57, 59
spectrum, v, vii, viii, 1, 4, 19, 24, 26, 28, 38, 39, 50, 57, 59, 61, 63, 74, 89, 94, 114, 120, 130, 132, 134, 135, 137, 138, 139, 162, 165, 166, 168, 170, 171, 173, 187, 188, 195, 197
stress, 48, 66, 67, 86, 88, 99, 123, 126, 139, 140, 141, 142, 143, 148, 149, 150, 155, 157, 164, 168, 169, 171, 190, 192, 196

Stroop color and word test (SCWT), vii, 1, 5, 28

symptom(s), v, vii, viii, 1, 2, 3, 4, 5, 7, 8, 9, 10, 12, 14, 15, 16, 18, 19, 20, 21, 22, 23, 24, 25, 26, 27, 28, 29, 30, 31, 36, 37, 40, 41, 43, 48, 55, 56, 62, 63, 64, 65, 66, 67, 68, 69, 70, 71, 73, 83, 87, 88, 90, 91, 94, 114, 118, 119, 131, 132, 134, 135, 140, 142, 143, 157, 158, 160, 173, 174, 176, 177, 180, 181, 182, 187, 188, 189, 190, 191

T

theory of mind, 36, 37, 38, 39, 44, 56, 57, 58, 59

therapy, vii, ix, 22, 39, 44, 55, 56, 58, 61, 68, 69, 70, 72, 73, 74, 77, 78, 79, 81, 82, 83, 86, 87, 96, 97, 98, 99, 100, 102, 103, 105, 107, 108, 111, 112, 127, 128, 129, 134, 136, 137, 138, 152, 154, 159, 161, 162, 164, 165, 166, 185, 187, 188, 189, 193, 194

transference, 79, 80

treatment and prevention, 62

treatment(s), vii, viii, 1, 9, 11, 13, 22, 35, 36, 37, 38, 41, 43, 44, 45, 48, 49, 50, 53, 55, 56, 57, 58, 62, 68, 69, 70, 71, 72, 79, 84, 87, 89, 95, 97, 98, 99, 100, 101, 105, 106, 107, 108, 109, 110, 111, 112, 113, 120, 123, 126, 127, 129, 130, 131, 132, 133, 134, 135, 136, 138, 140, 141, 142, 143, 148, 149, 159, 161, 162, 163, 164, 165, 172, 173, 181, 182, 188, 189, 190, 191, 192, 193, 194

trials, v, 6, 35

W

world federation for mental health (WFMH), viii, 62

wounds, ix, 78, 81, 82, 83